pn
11.6.08

Patient Care in Community Practice

Patient Care in Community Practice

A handbook of non-medicinal healthcare

Second edition

Edited by

Robin J Harman

PhD, MRPharmS

Independent Pharmaceutical and Regulatory Consultant
Farnham, Surrey, UK

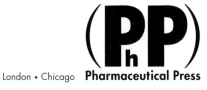

London • Chicago **Pharmaceutical Press**

Published by the Pharmaceutical Press
Publications division of the Royal Pharmaceutical Society of Great Britain

1 Lambeth High Street, London SE1 7JN, UK
100 South Atkinson Road, Suite 206, Grayslake, IL 60030-7820, USA

© Pharmaceutical Press 2002

First edition published 1989

Second edition published 2002

Text design by Barker/Hilsdon, Lyme Regis, Dorset
Typeset by Type Study, Scarborough, North Yorkshire
Printed in Great Britain by TJ International, Padstow, Cornwall

ISBN 0 85369 450 8

A catalogue record for this book is available from the British Library

To the memory of John Simpkins

Contents

Preface

It is now 13 years since the first edition of this book was published in 1989. The continued demand for the publication indicates that the desire for knowledge about this diverse range of conditions and products is as great as ever. This new edition includes details of all the latest developments in their treatment and management.

The objectives of this new edition of *Patient Care in Community Practice* remain the same as in the first: to provide a unique, single-volume, handy reference guide to the background, use and range of non-medicinal products and appliances that may be used in the home. The trend towards the management of as many conditions as possible in the home rather than in hospital has continued since the early 1990s. Hospital stays are as brief as is clinically possible, with patients returned into the care of practitioners in the community at a very early stage in the treatment of many conditions.

General practitioners, community pharmacists and district nurses have all had to adjust to the increased demands that this places on the primary healthcare team. For example, a patient who has undergone surgery that has resulted in the formation of a colostomy will invariably be home within five days of surgery (depending on the indication for the surgery). The onus is therefore laid on the primary healthcare services to manage the patient. This may include the selection and supply of dressings, the stoma appliance, and graduated compression hosiery for a non-ambulant patient, and dealing with special dietary requirements. Although this book is not a catalogue of the products available, it is intended to provide the background knowledge, and with it the confidence, that carers need to ensure that the patient's quality of life is maximised.

It is likely that the numbers of patients with the conditions described in this book will be small in comparison, for example, to the numbers undergoing antihypertensive therapy or requiring analgesic drugs, yet their very uncommonness renders the need for information all the more acute. In the UK, the *British National Formulary* (BNF) is the standard reference for all drug treatment, and almost all practitioners will be familiar with it. The *Nurse Prescriber's Formulary* describes those products that nurse practitioners can supply and gives more detailed information about some appliances (e.g. for stomas) than is possible within the BNF. The *Drug Tariff* lists all the appliances that can be supplied at NHS expense in England and Wales. Yet none of these excellent publications explains the rationale for the use and selection of non-medicinal products and appliances. This is the basis of the information provided in *Patient Care in Community Practice: A Handbook of Non-medicinal Healthcare*.

The other major change in the preparation of this new edition is that it is no longer a single-author publication. Each of the chapters has been written by an individual expert. Some of the revisions required have been limited: for example, there have not been many changes in the use or types of trusses available. In other topics the changes have been much greater, and this is reflected in the extent of the rewrite of individual chapters. There is also one new chapter that covers home enteral nutrition and complements those on dietary products and home parenteral nutrition.

The format for each chapter is to give an account of the condition(s) for which the products are used; this is followed by information about the range of products available, many of which are illustrated. Most chapters also include details of self-help organisations that practitioners may find beneficial, either to contact themselves or to whom they may wish to refer patients and/or their carers. Such organisations also provide a considerable amount of printed literature, supplemented by electronically available information on the internet. Indeed, the provision of so much information on the internet from these organisations and from manufacturers has been one of the most significant developments since the first edition of this book was published.

Chapter 1 details the causes, treatment and management of stomas. Emphasis is laid on the wide range of everyday problems about which ostomists may seek professional advice.

The management of urinary incontinence is an increasingly important aspect of healthcare, particularly in view of the increasing numbers of elderly people in the population. Chapter 2 discusses the causes and management of this potentially debilitating condition and highlights the diversity of aids and appliances available. The importance of selecting an appropriate device for patients and the criteria for that selection are described.

It is possible that the continued demand for 'low-tech' products such as trusses (Chapter 3) and graduated compression hosiery (Chapter

4) is a consequence of the delays in carrying out non-emergency surgery. Graduated compression hosiery is also commonly used postoperatively generally, and specifically pre- and postoperatively for varicose veins.

One area in which the greatest advances in our knowledge of the processes involved has occurred is that of wound healing, the complex process of which is described in Chapter 5. The range of products available for the different stages in the healing process continues to expand, and the latest information on these products is described.

The treatment of respiratory disorders in the home continues to develop. In Chapter 6 (Oxygen therapy), the use of oxygen cylinders is fully described. However, advances in the technology of oxygen concentrators are ongoing, resulting in their domestic use becoming more common. Technical advances have also been made in the products available for inhalation therapy (Chapter 7), with the objective of making their use as patient-friendly as possible. It is to be hoped that each improvement will enhance drug delivery and patient compliance.

Chapters 8, 9 and 10 are related, having as a common theme the use of special dietary products for the treatment of disease. In Chapter 8, the problems associated with malabsorption and intolerance conditions, and with errors of metabolism, are explained. Comprehensive details are given of the extensive range of products that can be used in the management of these conditions.

In Chapter 9, a description of the increasingly common home parenteral nutrition techniques is provided. Since its introduction in the 1960s, parenteral nutrition has been used in hospitals; the 1970s witnessed its introduction into the home. The highly technical nature of this form of treatment is stressed, and the problems that are likely to be encountered are outlined. The use of home parenteral nutrition is one example of the way in which patients can be safely managed in the much more 'normal' and friendly environment of their own home.

The use of home enteral nutrition (Chapter 10) is a logical extension of the use of home parenteral nutrition, and its use has grown rapidly since the early 1990s. It is now estimated that there are more people receiving home enteral nutrition in the community than in hospital. The techniques and the support that such patients will require in the community are explained in detail.

The causes and symptoms of end-stage renal disease are discussed in Chapter 11. Its management includes the use of dialysis in the home, and the techniques of continuous ambulatory peritoneal dialysis and haemodialysis are described. The ways in which practitioners in the community can assist in the management are also explained.

The book is illustrated with a comprehensive range of diagrams and photographs to assist in the identification and recognition of the types of products available. However, mention of such products is for illustrative purposes only and does not imply endorsement of those products.

The book does not seek to be a guide to all the items that may be prescribed at NHS expense in the UK. The current edition of the *Drug Tariff*, or other appropriate documents, should be consulted for this information.

Robin J Harman
March 2002

Acknowledgements

The production of this book has been made possible by the contributions of eight authors. I gratefully acknowledge their expertise in preparing this new edition.

Many of the authors have been assisted in the preparation of their chapters by manufacturers or other organisations. In particular, the help given by Cheryl Harrison at McCann Ericson Manchester in providing photographs for the chapter on graduated compression hosiery, and by Jean Acheson at Baxter Healthcare Ltd in providing photographs and background information for the chapter on dialysis at home, is gratefully acknowledged.

As in the previous edition of this book, some diagrams were drawn by John Simpkins, a friend and former colleague. It was therefore very poignant that John died during the preparation of this second edition and, in appreciation of his contribution and friendship, this book is dedicated to his memory.

About the editor

Robin J Harman PhD, MRPharmS has been an independent pharmaceutical and regulatory consultant since 1998, and has published extensively within the pharmaceutical and medical sectors. He is editor of
the second edition of the *Handbook of Pharmacy Health Education*
(London: Pharmaceutical Press, 2001). From 1990 to 1998 he was
Editor-in-Chief of *The Regulatory Affairs Journal* and *The Regulatory
Affairs Journal (Devices)*, which provide information to the pharmaceutical and medical devices industries, respectively. Previously, he was
an editor in the Department of Pharmaceutical Sciences at the Royal
Pharmaceutical Society of Great Britain. He edited the *Handbook of
Pharmacy Health-care: Diseases and Patient Advice* (London: Pharma-
ceutical Press, 1990), and authored the first edition of this book, *Patient
Care in Community Practice: A Handbook of Non-medicinal Healthcare* (London: Pharmaceutical Press, 1989).

Contributors

Sarah ME Cockbill PhD, LLM, MPharm, DAgVetPharm, MIPharmM, FCPP, FRPharmS
Senior Research Associate, Welsh School of Pharmacy, Cardiff

Derrick Garwood BDS
Medical Writer and Editorial Consultant, Royston, Hertfordshire

Eileen J Laughton PhD, MRPharmS
Freelance Medical Editor, Melton Mowbray, Leicestershire

Joanna Lumb FRPharmS
Medical Writer and Editor, London

Pamela Mason PhD, MRPharmS
Independent Pharmaceutical Consultant, London

Susan Shankie MSc, MRPharmS
Independent Pharmaceutical Consultant, Glasgow

Louise Whitley MSc, MRPharmS
Independent Pharmaceutical Consultant, Lyndhurst

Louise ME Wykes BSc
Royal Pharmaceutical Society of Great Britain, London

1

Stoma therapy

Susan Shankie

Approximately 100 000 people in the UK are living with a stoma at any one time, with approximately 18 000 new stomas being formed each year. With advances in surgical techniques, however, the number of people with a stoma has decreased over the last 10–15 years.

Definitions

Stoma (Gk. stoma = mouth)

An opening artificially produced for the removal of waste material from the body.

Colostomy

The colon is cut and brought to the surface of the body to form the stoma. The position of dissection of the colon has a significant effect on the nature of the stomal discharge or effluent.

Ileostomy

The ileum is cut and brought to the body's surface to form the stoma, usually as a consequence of complete removal of the colon.

Urostomy

Also known as ileal loop, ileal bladder or urinary conduit. The stoma is formed of a piece of isolated intestine (ileum or colon) into which the ureters are diverted.

Ureterostomy

A 'true' stoma is not formed, but the two ureters are brought directly to the surface of the body.

All patients who have a stoma are collectively described as 'ostomists'. The word 'ostomy' is frequently interchanged with 'stoma'.

Basic stoma formation

A piece of intestine with its blood supply and mesentery intact is brought through a hole in the abdominal wall. The gut is then turned back on itself to form a cuff, and the base of the cuff is stitched to the abdominal wall (Figure 1.1).

The stoma is reddish-pink, similar in colour to the inside of the mouth. Stomas that have a liquid or semiliquid discharge (Table 1.1) are sited proud of the surface of the abdomen to aid attachment of the collecting appliance. The mouth of the stoma usually remains closed unless material is being discharged from it, and the stoma will automatically shrink and dilate. Because of the absence of sensory nerves, the stoma is insensitive to touch, pressure and burning. Selection of a correctly fitting appliance is therefore essential. Badly fitting appliances will cause no physical discomfort to the ostomist but may produce irreversible damage to the stoma.

The formation of a stoma may be 'temporary' or 'permanent'.

Temporary stoma

A temporary stoma may also be termed a diverting stoma.

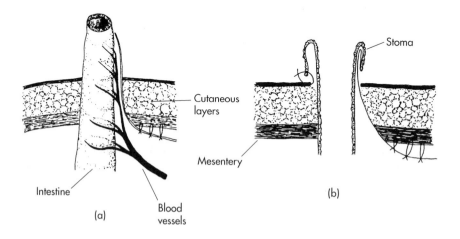

Figure 1.1 Formation of a stoma. (a) Protrusion of the length of intestine through the stomach wall. (b) Eversion of the piece of intestine to form the stoma.

Table 1.1 Permanent stomas

Type of ostomy	Nature of discharge	Frequency of discharge	Type of appliance usually required
Colostomy			
Descending	Solid (usually)	Intermittent	Non-drainable (closed)
Transverse	Formed and/or watery		
Ascending	Water or semisolid	Continuous	Drainable with wide spout
Ileostomy	Semiliquid containing digestive enzymes	Continuous	Drainable with wide spout
Urostomy	Urine	Continuous	Drainable with tap

Indications

The formation of a temporary stoma may be unplanned (e.g. as a result of a road traffic accident, or a shooting or stabbing). It may be carried out as elective surgery (e.g. before further surgery to provide an outlet for gastrointestinal contents while the distal portion of the intestine remains undisturbed). Common indications for elective temporary colostomy include diverticular disease, Hirschsprung's disease, and rectovaginal fistula. The integrity of the intestine may be restored once healing has taken place and normal gastrointestinal function resumed.

The two main types of temporary stoma, double-barrelled colostomy or loop ostomy, are outlined below.

Double-barrelled colostomy

A double-barrelled (Devine) colostomy may be necessary to relieve obstruction in the descending colon. Two stomas are formed, with the distal (or left) stoma remaining inactive (Figure 1.2). The proximal (right) stoma discharges the intestinal contents. The inactive stoma acts as an opening through which drugs may be passed to treat the condition in the distal intestine.

Loop ostomy

A section of intestine is brought out through the abdominal wall and is supported by a plastic bridge. Waste material is discharged through an

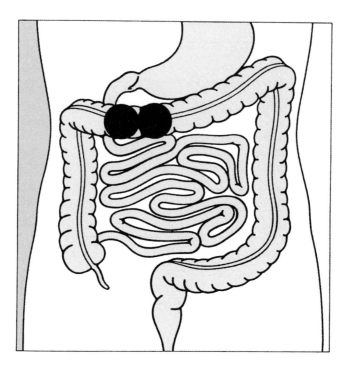

Figure 1.2 Double-barrelled (Devine) temporary colostomy.

incision in the outer-facing surface of the loop. A loop ostomy may be formed from a length of either ileum or colon.

Temporary stoma management

When the formation of a stoma is unplanned, the lack of opportunity to prepare the patient preoperatively may produce severe distress in addition to the distress caused by the trauma that necessitated the stoma formation. Full acceptance by ostomists of their new condition (even with the knowledge of its temporary nature) may be impossible.

Patients with a temporary stoma will have the colon and rectum still in place. Sometimes blood, mucus or faecal matter may be passed per rectum, which may be alarming for the patient but is quite normal.

The use of the term 'temporary' is relative. Patients may have such a stoma for periods of up to one year. Care of temporary stomas is as for permanent stomas and is described under the different stoma types.

Colostomy

Incidence and indications

Colostomists constitute the single largest group of ostomists and about 11 000 new colostomies are formed annually. The commonest indications are:

- cancer of the colon, rectum and anus
- rectal prolapse
- severe trauma, where temporary colostomy is not feasible
- an irreparably damaged spinal cord.

The extent of the disease or damage to the large intestine determines the external position of the stoma and the nature of its discharge, and thus the type of appliance required (Table 1.1).

Descending colostomy

This is the most common type of colostomy. The stoma is formed from the descending colon and the proximal colon is retained intact (Figure 1.3). Considerable amounts of fluid may be reabsorbed from waste material during its passage along the colon. Consequently, once the stoma has settled down postoperatively, the discharge from the stoma is usually solidly formed and virtually free of digestive enzymes. Because the discharge is solidly formed, a closed bag (i.e. non-drainable) can be used. Depending on preoperative bowel habits, control of the timing of discharge may be possible and in a small minority of patients the use of a complete appliance may not be necessary: a stoma cap or small activity pouch (mini bag) may be used instead.

Transverse colostomy

This type of stoma is formed from a length of transverse colon and is often a temporary measure. Because the stoma is formed much higher up the intestine than a descending colostomy, the effluent is more fluid and less regularly discharged. A bag is therefore required. The type of bag depends on the frequency and consistency of the effluent: a drainable bag may be used that is changed every three to four days; alternatively, a non-drainable bag may be used that is changed daily.

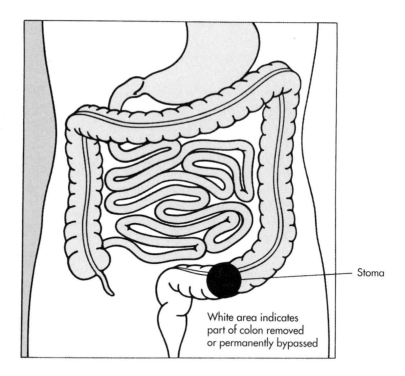

Stoma

White area indicates
part of colon removed
or permanently bypassed

Figure 1.3 Descending colostomy.

Ascending colostomy

This is not a common type of stoma. The removal of almost all of the large intestine permits only minimal fluid absorption, and the stomal discharge is liquid or paste-like and flows continuously, thus requiring the use of a drainable bag. Management of an ascending colostomy is essentially the same as that of an ileostomy (*see* Ileostomy management, below). Because the effluent contains digestive enzymes, skin protection is important with this type of stoma.

Colostomy management

Most patients with a new permanent colostomy are over 55 years of age and may find it more difficult than younger patients to adapt to their new condition. In addition, the presence of other conditions (e.g. reduced manual dexterity and reduced vision) may complicate management.

Diet

All healthy individuals with 'normal' bowel function may associate particular foods with changes in bowel action, and they may make conscious decisions to avoid such foods. Colostomists are no different in this respect. They should be encouraged to maintain as varied a diet as possible to ensure adequate nutrition, and they should note which foods produce a change in the nature of stomal discharge. These foods do not have to be avoided, but consumption in moderation is advised.

Diarrhoea may be caused by:

Beans	Raw fruit	Soup
Peas	Cauliflower	Spices
Excess beer or lager	Cabbage	Prunes
Spinach	Chocolate	

Foods must be completely disintegrated, as the colostomist cannot exert mental control over evacuation and stomal blockage may develop. All ostomists should be advised to chew food thoroughly before swallowing. Foods that may cause blockage include:

• seed-containing foods (e.g. tomatoes and pomegranates)
• high-fibre foods (e.g. wholemeal bread)
• cabbage, celery, cauliflower and coconut.

Constipation may be caused by insufficient fluid intake, by vegetables, and by cooked fruits.

Any advice about diet must stress the importance of maintaining a balanced diet that fulfils the body's nutritional requirements, and at the same time must take into account the patient's domestic and financial situation.

It is important to bear in mind that changes in discharge may also be caused by a recurrence of the underlying disease process that led to the stoma formation.

Odour

The choice of foods will affect the degree of odour of the discharge. Foods that appear to worsen this problem include:

Baked beans	Some cheeses	Onions
Fish	Strawberries	Asparagus
Eggs	Cabbage	Beer

A reduction in the odour of the faeces has been noted following the ingestion of natural yoghurt and buttermilk.

Flatus

As food passes along the colon its bacterial decomposition may generate gases. A patient with a descending colostomy may have a more severe flatus problem than a patient with an ascending colostomy. Flatus may also be more of a problem in the initial stages, and sometimes for up to a year after bowel surgery. Eating small, frequent meals can ease the problem, as can eating slowly. Foods that cause a significant increase in flatus include:

Baked beans	Greens	Beer
Fizzy drinks	Onions	Highly spiced foods (e.g. curries)

A regular and varied diet may help to reduce the problem.

Irrigation

Colostomy irrigation is an alternative to natural evacuation that may be suitable for some people. The significant advantage of irrigation over normal bowel evacuation is that irrigation is only needed about every 24 or 48 hours. In the intervening periods a stoma cap can be substituted for a complete appliance (see below). Dietary restrictions can also be relaxed, as the production of flatus and odour is minimised.

The irrigation process involves instilling 1–1.5 L of warm water (25–30°C) over about 20 minutes via a catheter into the stoma until the distal colon is filled. The presence of water in the intestine induces peristalsis, causing the fluid to be discharged from the stoma through a spout into the toilet. The complete process takes about one hour and is suitable only for healthy and competent colostomists (ideally those with a descending colostomy) with a stoma that discharges formed stools. The procedure is not suitable for elderly, arthritic or partially sighted patients, or for patients with stomal abnormalities or whose stoma produces soft, unformed stools. To ensure its correct use, 'starter' irrigation sets are only available from hospitals, although replacement parts may be ordered through community pharmacies.

Ileostomy

Incidence and indications

About 2500 ileostomies are formed each year in England and Wales. The most common indications are ulcerative colitis and Crohn's disease unresponsive to drug therapy, although familial polyposis coli and cancer of the colon and rectum may also be causative conditions.

Ulcerative colitis is inflammation and ulceration of the colon, always involving the rectum. The common presenting symptoms include diarrhoea, accompanied by pus and mucus in the stool. Blood may be lost faecally, resulting in anaemia. Arthritis and other inflammatory disorders may accompany colitis.

Crohn's disease is a chronic form of inflammation of the gastro-intestinal wall that may affect any part of the gastrointestinal tract. In Crohn's disease and ulcerative colitis emergency surgery may be required, but the formation of an ileostomy is normally a planned procedure.

Conventional ileostomy

A traditional operation to form an ileostomy involves removal of the entire length of the large bowel, including the rectal stump (Figure 1.4).

One modification is Park's technique, in which the short length of rectum is retained intact. At a later stage it may be possible to construct a pouch in place of the large intestine (an ileoanal pouch), rejoining the end of the ileum to the rectum. As a result, conventional excretion of faeces may be resumed.

Continent (Kock's) ileostomy

A conventional ileostomy discharges intestinal contents continuously. In contrast, the output from a Kock ileostomy is intended to collect in a sac or reservoir formed within the abdomen. A catheter can be inserted through a reversible valve to empty the contents of the sac several times a day. In theory, an appliance need be worn only intermittently. In practice, however, the integrity of the valve in the abdominal wall cannot be guaranteed, and the leakage of intestinal contents through the valve may necessitate the continuous use of an appliance. This procedure is less popular since the introduction of the ileoanal pouch procedure.

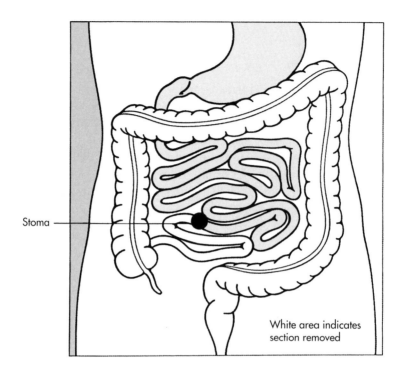

Stoma

White area indicates
section removed

Figure 1.4 Ileostomy.

Ileostomy management

Compared to new colostomists, most new ileostomists are relatively young (20–30 years of age). They may therefore adapt much more readily to their new condition than older patients. Another significant factor in assisting ileostomists to come to terms with their condition is the contrast with their previously restricted lifestyle, in which an inflammatory bowel condition prevented them from moving far from a toilet. The formation of an ileostomy produces a significant improvement in health and quality of life, greatly facilitating adaptation.

The effluent from an ileostomy flows more or less continuously (see Table 1.1) and is usually liquid, or sometimes a semisolid paste. A drainable bag is therefore required that may be left in place for three to five days and which may require draining about five times a day.

General ileostomy management is similar to colostomy management in respect of diet, odour and flatus (see above). Potential problems in ileostomy management arise from the increased loss of fluid and electrolytes, and from the presence of digestive proteolytic enzymes in the discharge that can cause skin problems.

Fluid loss

In normal intestinal function the amount of fluid lost in the faeces is about 100–150 mL. Absorption of sodium and chloride ions takes place in the colon in exchange for potassium and bicarbonate ions. Thus, in the presence of an ileostomy the facility for fluid and electrolyte exchange is significantly reduced. Loss of fluid may result in dehydration, which may be accompanied by decreased urine output. Ileostomists must therefore compensate for increased fluid and electrolyte loss in their intake. They should be advised to drink an extra 500–800 mL each day and to add salt to all meals.

Kidney stone formation

The combination of reduced urine formation and increased loss of sodium ions may produce metabolic acidosis, together with an increased risk of uric acid stone formation. Increased fluid intake (as described above) may reduce this risk.

Gallstone formation

Disruption of the enterohepatic circulation in terminal ileum loss may lead to gallstone formation as a result of inadequate distribution of bile salts. This can be a significant problem in ileostomy management. Replacement therapy with bile acids (e.g. chenodeoxycholic acid) is contraindicated as it produces severe diarrhoea.

Urostomy

Incidence and indications

About 2000 urostomies are formed annually in England and Wales, and an estimated 11 000 patients currently have this type of stoma.

The two primary indications for urostomy formation are:

- failure of bladder function owing to interference with nervous control or to the presence of a congenital lesion (e.g. spina bifida)
- bladder removal, commonly as a result of carcinoma.

In spina bifida the vertebral arches fail to close, exposing the contents of the spinal canal. If the intact meninges herniate through the bony lesion, a meningomyelocele may be formed. Rupture of the sac, together with nerve damage, leads to disruption of motor and sensory nerve function below the lesion. Urinary incontinence (see also Chapter 2) may arise through effects on bladder function and require the formation of a urostomy, although the use of intermittent self-catheterisation is gaining popularity as an alternative.

Spina bifida patients with a urostomy are commonly young (less than 20 years of age); patients with bladder cancer may be middle-aged or elderly.

Urostomy formation

This procedure is also termed a urinary diversion. One stoma only is formed from a section of colon or, more commonly, ileum. The ureters are diverted into the piece of gut, which then acts as a channel (conduit) for urinary discharge (Figure 1.5). It was originally hoped that the piece of intestine would act as a reservoir from which the urine could be occasionally voided (hence the former term, ileal bladder), but in

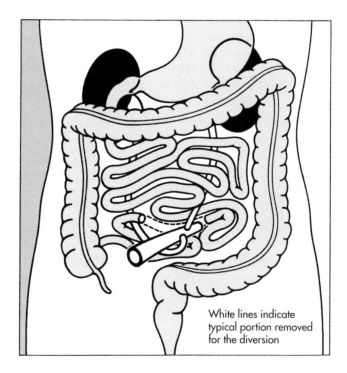

White lines indicate typical portion removed for the diversion

Figure 1.5 Urostomy.

practice the urine drains continuously from the stoma. Normal intestinal function is restored once the section has been removed to form the conduit.

An alternative to the formation of a urostomy is an operation to produce a ureterostomy. In this surgical procedure the two ureters are brought to the surface of the body to form two urinary stomas, one each side of the midline. Problems associated with the concurrent management of two appliances, and the much-increased risk of transfer of infection from one kidney to the other, have greatly reduced the usefulness of this procedure. Sometimes the two ureters may be joined together and brought to the surface to form one stoma.

Urostomy management

A urostomy discharges urine continuously, requiring a drainable bag with a tap (see Table 1.1). As urine is ammoniacal it will damage skin, and it is therefore important to avoid leakages and ensure adequate skin protection. Fluid intake is also an important part of urostomy management.

The segment of ileum or colon used to form a urostomy continues to secrete mucus. Patients should therefore be warned that it is normal for their urine to contain some mucus; this may diminish over time.

Fluid intake

To minimise the risk of infection and prevent stasis of urine, urostomists must be advised to increase their daily fluid intake to about 2–3 L per 24 hours. However, unless adequate toilet facilities are available, too great an increase should also be avoided. There is an increased risk of leakage from the appliance when it is full or nearly full.

Urinary odour

Urinary odour, especially when accompanied by cloudiness of the urine, generally indicates the presence of infection. The odour is produced by the presence of breakdown products of nitrogenous materials. This symptom may be partially reduced by increasing the fluid intake, but the underlying source of the infection should be sought and remedied. Elimination of infection is particularly important when the urostomy is formed because of the absence or removal of the bladder, as infection may rapidly ascend to the kidneys.

The only food that has been associated with the presence of urinary odour is asparagus. Odour from any source may be reduced if fruit juices are drunk to render the urine more acidic. This precaution may also help to reduce the likelihood of infection.

Appliance information

Each type of stoma requires a different type of appliance (see Table 1.1). The design of stoma appliances has progressed significantly over the last few years, partly because of the development of new plastic materials. The wide range of equipment available allows patients to select appliances that suit them individually. Ensuring that patients choose the most appropriate equipment can do much to enhance their quality of life. Ostomists will have confidence in an appliance if it is:

- leakproof
- odour-proof
- rustle-proof and unobtrusive
- easy to empty and change
- of adequate capacity
- comfortable to wear.

Table 1.2 gives an indication of the range of appliances and accessories that are available and some of the details that are needed for ordering supplies. Further details are provided in the text below; it is not intended to provide comprehensive information on the entire range of commercially available appliances. In England and Wales, comprehensive information can be found in the current edition of the *Drug Tariff*, Part IXC.

Regularly required items

The bag

Bags are also known as pouches. Bags for all types of stoma fall into two categories: one-piece or two-piece appliances. One-piece appliances incorporate a means of attaching the device to the body (i.e. a base-plate or flange) that is integral with the bag. Two-piece appliances consist of a flange that attaches to the peristomal skin. The bag, which comes separately, then clips on to this flange and allows the bag to be changed without disturbing the peristomal skin. The flange can be left in place for several days.

Table 1.2 Range of stoma appliances and accessories available

Item	Details	Additional information required
Regularly required items		
Bag	Manufacturer	
	Type of bag	Non-drainable/drainable
		One-piece/two-piece
		With or without flatus filter
	Flange type	Standard or convex
	Material of construction	Clear/opaque
	Size/capacity	Small/medium/large
	Stoma diameter	Specified in mm (or starter hole)
Infrequently required items		
Belt	Waist size	Usually available adjustable
	Pressure plate	Separate or integral with appliance
Optional items		
Peristomal skin wafer/washer (where not an integral part of the appliance)	Manufacturer	Standard/extra thin
Adhesive	Type	Tape/solution/spray
Night-drainage system	For urostomy use	Must be compatible with appliance used
Stoma caps	For colostomy use	
Bag covers	Plain/patterned	
Skin adhesive removers	Type	Liquid/spray
Deodorants	Type	Liquid/powder/spray
Skin protectives and fillers	Type	
Convex inserts	Manufacturer	

Bags may be closed (i.e. non-drainable, Figure 1.6), drainable through a wide neck (for semiliquid or liquid effluent) with a clip fastening (Figure 1.7), or drainable through a tap (for urine, Figure 1.8).

Appliances are attached to the body by the flange. Modern flanges are made from hard, soft, semirigid or flexible material and usually have an inner protective area (the peristomal skin wafer) and an outer adhesive area. On modern appliances these adhesives and skin wafers are hypoallergenic and resistant to breakdown by intestinal contents or urine. Some appliances include the skin wafer only or the adhesive area only. Adhesives and skin wafers are available separately for those patients requiring them (see below). Convex flanges are available for patients with a retracted or awkwardly sited stoma (see also Convex inserts, below). The older 'traditional' flanges are non-adhesive and may be retained using a belt. They may be made from a variety of materials (e.g. foam, rubber, latex and plastic). Their use has largely been superseded by the modern flanges.

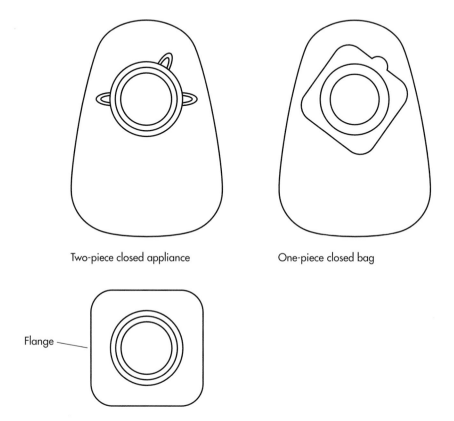

Two-piece closed appliance   One-piece closed bag

Flange

Figure 1.6 Examples of closed (non-drainable) appliances.

Ostomists with a well-formed colostomy discharge may not require any adhesive; the bag is kept in place using a belt and belt attachment or pressure plate (see below). Adhesive is essential for stomas with a more liquid discharge, to prevent leakage.

Closed bags usually incorporate a flatus filter to allow the release of gases and prevent ballooning of the bag. The filter usually incorporates a carbon/charcoal component that absorbs odours. Self-adhesive filters are also available separately. Filter covers or stickers are available that allow the filters to be inactivated. For example, if only a little flatus

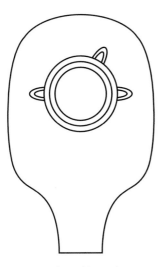
Two-piece drainable appliance

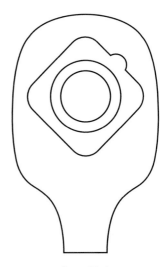
One-piece drainable bag

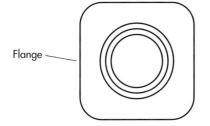
Flange

Figure 1.7 Examples of drainable appliances (wide neck).

is passed the sides of the bag can stick to each other, preventing any discharged stool from dropping down into the pouch (sometimes called 'pancaking'). Drainable bags do not usually have filters, as the liquid effluent would block the filter. Flatus can easily be removed by opening the clip on the bag. Flatus may also be released from a two-piece system by unclipping the bag from the flange.

Traditionally, reusable black or white rubber appliances were the only bags available. They had the advantage of opacity, but on continued use they absorbed faecal and urinary odour. Although some of these products are still available, their use has been largely superseded by the development of disposable plastic appliances. Plastic appliances are light and unobtrusive, and improvements in their manufacture have led to the development of bags that are guaranteed to be almost 100% leakproof.

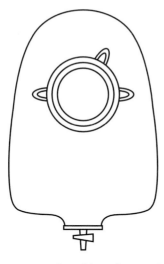
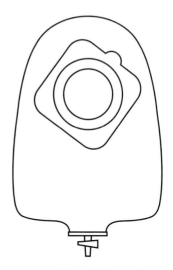

Two-piece drainable appliance with tap   One-piece drainable bag with tap

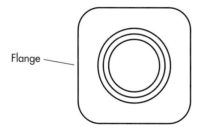

Flange

Figure 1.8 Examples of urostomy appliances.

They may be transparent or opaque. Transparent bags are used in the immediate postoperative period to allow easy inspection of the stoma and its effluent. Thereafter, opaque bags are generally preferred.

Sometimes plastic bags can rustle under clothing, making the wearer self-conscious about their presence. Many of the most recently developed plastic bags have soft cover materials that reduce the rustling and reduce the moisture that develops behind the bag.

Bags are ordered by volume of bag required and also by size of opening to fit around the stoma. They generally come in small, medium and large sizes to suit different amounts of effluent and for overnight use. A mini size is also available that may be used when extra discretion is particularly required (e.g. during swimming). Bags also come in a paediatric size.

Measuring cards are available for accurate assessment of the correct size of bag opening required. Remeasuring is essential during the period immediately after surgery as the diameter of the stoma may alter as the intestine settles down. If the opening is too large discharge may seep on to the peristomal skin, causing excoriation. Conversely, as the stoma possesses no sensory nerve endings, serious damage may occur before it is realised that the bag opening is too small. Precut circular openings are available. For patients with an irregular shaped stoma, flanges with a small starter hole are used that allow any shape or size to be cut.

A stoma plug

This may be inserted into the stoma of a descending colostomy that is producing regular, firm stools. It is not suitable for a colostomy patient whose bowel action is loose, or for ileostomists or urostomists. The portion inside the stoma consists of a column of soft, flexible foam covered in a water-soluble film. When the plug is inserted into the stoma, the film dissolves and the foam expands to fill the channel. The expanded plug prevents the passage of faeces, but allows flatus to escape through an integral filter and vent. The plug may remain in position for up to 12 hours and need only be removed to allow the passage of faeces.

Infrequently required items

Belt

Many modern appliances incorporate an integral attachment for a belt. A separate pressure plate may be required if attachments are not integral. Belts may be used to secure a non-adhesive appliance in place, or some people using an appliance with an adhesive prefer to use a belt in addition to provide extra security. Pharmacists should be aware that belt attachments for appliances from different manufacturers are not interchangeable. The use of a belt may assist in keeping the bag in position, especially when the downward pressure from the bag increases as it fills. Belts may be one size, or may be ordered according to the waist measurement of the patient. They are usually made of elastic. A 'belt' may also be in the form of a support garment, such as an ostomy girdle or panty brief that incorporates a hole over the stoma area.

Optional items

Peristomal skin wafer

This is a protective layer formed of Stomahesive®, Cohesive®, karaya, or of a fabric support collar around a central wafer. It is used to protect the delicate peristomal skin from both adhesive and effluent. Peristomal skin wafers may or may not be incorporated into an appliance. If the peristomal skin wafer does not form an integral part of the appliance, separate units may be used to which the appliance may be attached. In each case, the hole in the centre of the wafer must be cut to the correct size, using a measuring guide.

Adhesive

Many appliances used nowadays incorporate an adhesive. However, a wide range of adhesives is available separately for those patients who prefer to use a non-adhesive appliance. Adhesives may also be used by patients with 'difficult' stomas who find the adhesion produced by the adhesive incorporated into the device insufficient. The adhesives available include hypoallergenic adhesive tapes, adhesive discs, rings, pads and plasters. These are commonly double-sided adhesive products that are attached to the skin on one side and the bag on the other. If greater adhesiveness is needed, pastes, sprays and solutions can be applied. To minimise the risks of allergic reactions and skin damage occurring when the adhesive is removed, these products should be used carefully.

Night-drainage systems

As the flow of urine from a urostomy is continuous, the use of night-drainage appliances (Figure 1.9) may encourage confident undisturbed sleep. A night-time drainage tube may be automatically supplied with urostomy bags. Some manufacturers may also supply a bag (of up to 2 L capacity).

Stoma caps

A stoma cap may be worn instead of a bag by patients with a descending colostomy whose bowel movements are predictable. A cap may also be worn for short periods (e.g. during sport and swimming) or by patients whose bowel activity is regulated by irrigation.

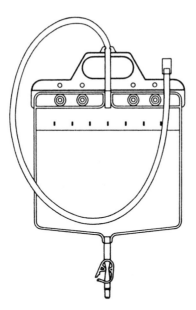

Figure 1.9 Urinary night-drainage system.

Bag covers

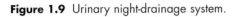

Plain or patterned bag covers are available in a wide range of materials (e.g. cotton, linen and Lycra) and may be useful for increasing the confidence of patients who may feel that their appliance or stoma is visible through thin clothing. They may also be useful in preventing discomfort caused by the bag clinging to the skin, leading to perspiration and, in some cases, rashes.

Adhesive removers

Liquid or spray adhesive removers may be necessary to remove residual adhesive that may prevent the satisfactory fitting of a new appliance. These adhesive removers are formulated specifically for ostomists to minimise skin irritation, although they should still be used with caution. Ostomists should be advised not to use adhesive removers that have not been formulated for use with stomas.

Deodorants

Deodorants in drop or powder form may be added to a bag before it is fitted to neutralise the odour of the discharge. They are generally used only in older appliances, as the modern systems are odour-proof if fitted correctly. Deodorant atomisers may be useful when the appliance is being changed or emptied.

Skin fillers and protectives

Many patients (especially older ostomists) may be overweight and possess significant folds of abdominal skin. As a result, it may be virtually impossible to attach an appliance effectively and with confidence. Skin fillers consisting of pastes, powders or gels may be useful in obtaining as smooth a surface as possible on which to place the appliance.

Barrier creams, lotions and wipes may be effective in limiting excoriation around the stoma, especially if the bag is changed frequently. However, great care in their use is essential to ensure that the skin is not left greasy, thereby preventing adhesion of the appliance.

Washers

Some stomas have a hollow area encircling the stoma that makes adequate attachment of a bag very difficult. Washers (circular rings made from hydrocolloid or karaya), also known as seals, may be used to build up this hollow area to allow better appliance attachment.

Convex inserts

Stomas that lie flush with the skin, retracted stomas, or stomas sited in a skin fold may require a convex insert to obtain a satisfactory bag fit. The convex insert fits into the appliance and forces the bag flange into a convex shape that improves the contact between the flange and the skin, forming a more secure fit.

Clips

Spare clips can be ordered for drainable bags. These may be in the form of rigid plastic or soft wire.

Bridges

When some appliances become warm the plastic of the stoma bag tends to close in on itself, forming a vacuum and preventing the discharge dropping into the bag. Stoma bridges are used to prevent this happening.

Practicalities of appliance use

Changing the appliance

With the possible exception of an established stoma formed from a descending colon, stomal discharge is usually unregulated. The appliance should be changed before eating or drinking (e.g. early in the morning) to reduce the quantity of discharge, which may interfere with changing. The following guidelines for changing may be used:

- Remove the appliance. If it is attached to the skin by adhesive, removal should be done carefully to minimise skin damage. The appliance should be removed from the top downwards, following the line of hair growth.
- Wash the skin with warm water. Some patients may prefer to use soap as well, to add to the feeling of cleanliness. Non-perfumed soap should be used and it must be rinsed off thoroughly. Adhesive removers may be necessary to clean the skin, but sensitivity to these agents may occur.
- Dry the peristomal skin, preferably by patting rather than rubbing. Tissue should be used rather than cotton wool that sheds fibres.
- Occasionally peristomal hair may require removal. This should ideally be done with an electric, not a wet, razor. Great care must be taken during shaving as the insensitive stoma will bleed easily. If bleeding persists or derives from within the stoma, medical advice should be sought urgently.
- Fit a new appliance according to manufacturer's instructions. This may be best achieved with the patient lying flat or standing. Sitting may produce folds in the skin that will stretch on standing, reducing the attachment of the appliance.
- If air is present in the appliance after fixing, it should be removed by opening the tap or clip (on a drainable appliance) or forcing it through the flatus filter (on a closed appliance).

Drainage

To drain an appliance, patients can sit or stand over the toilet. Colostomy patients with a drainable or non-drainable appliance should empty the bag or change it after each movement. The continuous nature of the discharge from an ileostomy or urostomy precludes frequent changes, and the bag should be emptied when it becomes more than half full.

Bowel activity is much reduced at night, and an ileostomist may be able to change to a smaller appliance overnight. Urostomy action remains constant and night-drainage systems are available (see above) to avoid repeated awakenings to empty the appliance.

Disposal

Most modern appliances are made of plastic, and after they have been emptied and rinsed can only be destroyed satisfactorily by incineration. However, this is not practical for most ostomists, and one of the following methods should be used:

- Wrap the empty appliance in paper or newspaper, fold securely and place it in the dustbin. Plastic disposal sacks are also available.
- Collection by the local Department of Environmental Health can be arranged. However, this may embarrass patients as it draws attention to their condition.

There are a few completely disposable bags available that may be flushed down the toilet. However, care must be taken with the type of toilet used for disposal. Ostomists must be advised not to dispose of other types of bag down the toilet.

Skin problems

In all types of ostomy, dermatitis caused by the discharge or by the proximity of the appliance to the skin may damage the peristomal skin.

Dermatitis caused by the discharge from the stoma may arise through a poorly fitting appliance, leakage from the appliance, or a poorly sited stoma. The interaction between the discharge and the skin is a particular problem with an ileostomy (owing to the presence of proteolytic enzymes) and a urostomy (because of the presence of ammoniacal products). Colostomy discharge is less detrimental to the skin.

Stoma size should be remeasured periodically to ensure the appliance fits well and to avoid skin irritation caused by poor fitting. Remeasurement is especially important in the initial months following stoma formation, as stoma size will alter during this period. If leakage occurs, it may be because of an uneven surface for appliance attachment or scars from previous surgical operations, and it may be extremely difficult to overcome.

Dermatitis may be provoked by a hypersensitivity reaction between the skin and the appliance, adhesive agents, or cleaning agents, or a combination of all three. Since the advent of modern plastic appliances and hypoallergenic adhesives these problems have significantly decreased. However, reactions may still occur and it is important to distinguish between those caused by the discharge and those provoked by the appliance. As a general rule, dermatitis caused by the discharge produces a generalised erythema, whereas that caused by the appliance may develop only at the areas of contact between the skin and the appliance. Bag covers (see above) may help in reducing skin reactions to constituents of the plastic appliances. Too-frequent bag changes can cause skin problems.

Skin problems are notoriously difficult to eradicate and may be responsible for a significant reduction in the quality of life of the ostomist. Topical creams and ointments should be avoided, as they may reduce the adhesiveness of the appliance and thereby perpetuate the problem.

The use of karaya gum washers or peristomal wafers, or both, may be the only satisfactory solution to the problem. Once the condition has improved, it is imperative to prevent its recurrence by eliminating the cause.

Factors affecting the quality of life

Employment

The successful rehabilitation of ostomists in employment may enhance their acceptance of their condition. Most ostomists can return to their former employment, with the possible exception of those in occupations that involve heavy lifting or straining of abdominal muscles. Some employers may require convincing that the presence of an ostomy will have little effect on the work performance of the individual. In young patients the formation of a stoma may significantly improve their general health and lead to much greater productivity.

Domestic and family relationships

For young children, the complete involvement of the parents pre- and postoperatively is essential. Teachers should be advised of the presence of the ostomy to speed the complete reintegration of the young ostomist in normal activities.

In adolescence and young adulthood, relationships with the opposite sex must be approached realistically. Total concealment of the appliance is usually impossible, especially when it has become full. Only by experience will the young ostomist be able to judge the best time to tell their partner of their condition. With an understanding partner, honesty is always the best policy.

For patients whose ostomy is formed within marriage, its total acceptance by the spouse is essential but is not always automatic. Accepting that a period of adjustment is essential for both partners may lessen the risk of estrangement.

Impotence and incontinence may develop postoperatively; vaginal damage may also occur, leading to pelvic sepsis. These effects may require special counselling. To some ostomists the 'disfigurement' of their body by the stoma could be worsened by their inability to have 'normal' sexual relationships.

Pregnancy

Anatomically, pregnancy may be feasible for ostomists and is frequently successful. Women are normally advised, however, to wait at least two years after surgery before considering pregnancy. Precautions against iron deficiency and megaloblastic anaemias taken in a normal pregnancy must be especially stringent in an ostomy pregnancy, particularly for an ileostomist. Intravenous or intramuscular administration of iron preparations may be necessary.

If abdominal colic occurs, the ileostomist should be referred for confirmation of uninterrupted intestinal flow.

Displacement, enlargement, prolapse or retraction of the stoma may occur during confinement, but patients should be reassured that automatic correction usually occurs after birth. The position and state of the stoma should be monitored and appliances revised as appropriate.

Sport

Sporting activities can usually be resumed after a postoperative recuperation period, and these may assist in the rehabilitation of the ostomist. Only those sports which are potentially harmful (e.g. boxing, wrestling, karate) should be excluded, and contact sports (e.g. rugby and football) should be undertaken with care.

Alcohol

Social intake of alcohol may be considered acceptable provided no other factors (e.g. prescribed medicines) indicate otherwise. A high level of urinary throughput is essential in a urostomy, but this should not be achieved with alcohol (e.g. beer), as the consequent dehydration may increase the risk of infection.

Travel

When the ostomist is driving, the seat belt may lie across the appliance or the stoma, or both, generating increased pressure within the appliance. This may be partially relieved by the use of a peg or clip on the cross-strap of the seat belt, which slightly reduces its pressure under normal circumstances but does not interfere with the effectiveness of the device in an emergency. Compliance with current legislation is essential. The ostomist should bear in mind that it is generally easier to refashion a stoma than to rebuild a scarred face.

Air travel may pose problems. Inflation of the bag may occur at reduced cabin pressures, increasing the risks of leakage. Spare appliances should always be carried in the hand luggage. The limited toilet facilities on aircraft may cause the ostomist concern. Regulation of diet or fluid intake before the flight may be advisable.

Drugs

Drug administration may lead to changes in bowel activity in all members of the population. The effects of these changes may be especially pronounced for the colostomist and ileostomist.

Drugs that possess anticholinergic activity (e.g. antihistamines, tricyclic antidepressants, certain drugs used in parkinsonism, and antipsychotic drugs) may lead to constipation. Opioid analgesics may exert a similar effect. Calcium- or aluminium-containing antacids can also produce constipation in patients with a colostomy. Conversely, more severe problems in management of the colostomy and ileostomy may be caused by agents that produce diarrhoea (e.g. adrenergic neurone-blocking drugs and antibiotics). Magnesium-containing antacids can produce diarrhoea in the patient with an ileostomy. Iron preparations may also cause loose stools.

Drugs that affect electrolyte and fluid balance (e.g. diuretics and antacids) should be used with caution, especially with an ileostomy. Calcium-containing antacids can lead to urinary calculi formation in patients with a urostomy.

Some types of formulation may be inappropriate for the ostomist because of the reduced surface area available for absorption.

Sustained-release preparations may be excreted through an ileostomy or a colostomy before they have dissolved. Enteric-coated preparations, in which the formulated drug must pass to the alkaline environment of the small intestine before dissolution, are usually totally ineffective in the ileostomist and only partially effective in the colostomist.

A female ileostomist should be advised to consider methods of contraception other than the pill, which may be ineffective as oral contraceptives are absorbed high up in the small intestine.

The colour of the faeces or urine may change in patients prescribed a varied range of drugs. Patients should be reassured that the discoloration is expected and does not reflect abnormal changes in the functioning of their stoma. Table 1.3 indicates some of the colour changes that may occur.

Table 1.3 Colour changes produced in stools and urine by drugs

Colour	Drug
Colour of stools	
Blackened	Bismuth and iron salts
	Charcoal
Pink to red to black	Phenylbutazone
	Salicylates
	Oral anticoagulants
	Heparin
Green or green-grey	Antibiotics
	Indometacin
White, grey or flecked	Antacids
Colour of urine[a]	
Brown/rusty yellow	Chloroquine
	Nitrofurantoin
	Senna
Red/brown	Anthraquinones
	Metronidazole
	Phenothiazines
	Rifampicin
Green or green-blue	Amitriptyline
	Indometacin
	Sulphonamides
	Triamterene
Orange	Dantron
	Warfarin

[a]The colour may vary considerably with the degree of diuresis.

Current information on the use of drugs in stoma patients may be found in the *British National Formulary*.

The role of the pharmacist

Ostomists are entirely reliant on their appliances to be capable of leading a relatively normal life. Patients may obtain their appliances from community pharmacists or by mail order from various suppliers. Pharmacists can do much to gain the confidence of the ostomist by keeping records of each patient's supplies and ensuring that adequate stocks are held at the time that a prescription for stoma equipment is presented. Having gained the patient's confidence, the pharmacist (perhaps in conjunction with the local stoma care nurse) will be in a position to advise the ostomist of ways to improve his or her quality of life. The pharmacist is also ideally placed to detect early signs of problems. As the ostomist ages their requirements may gradually change. The pharmacist will be able to suggest suitable modifications to their regimens.

Further reading

Breeze J (2000). Stoma care – an update. *Pharm J* 265: 823–826.

Roberts J McH, Singleton M, Adair CG (1994). *Stoma Care: A Self-study Course for Pharmacists*. Belfast: Northern Ireland Centre for Postgraduate Pharmaceutical Education and Training.

Taylor P, ed. (1999). *Stoma Care in the Community: A Clinical Resource for Practitioners*. London: Nursing Times Books.

Useful addresses

Association for Spina Bifida and Hydrocephalus (ASBAH)
ASBAH House
42 Park Road
Peterborough PE1 2UQ
Tel: 01733 555988

British Colostomy Association
15 Station Road
Reading
Berkshire RG1 1LG
Tel: 0800 3284257 *or* 0118 9391537
www.bcass.org.uk

Ileostomy and Internal Pouch Support Group
National Office
PO Box 132
Scunthorpe
North Lincs DN15 9YW
Tel: 0800 0184724 *or* 01724 720150
www.ileostomypouch.demon.co.uk

National Advisory Service for Parents of Children with a Stoma
(NASPCS)
51 Anderson Drive
Valley View Park
Darvel
Ayrshire KA17 0DE
Tel: 01560 322024

National Association for Colitis and Crohn's Disease
4 Beaumont House
Sutton Road
St. Albans
Herts AL1 5HH
Tel: 01727 844296 *or* 01727 830038
www.nacc.org.uk

Urostomy Association
Buckland
Beaumont Park
Danbury
Essex CM3 4DE
Tel: 01245 224294
www.uagbi.org

2

Management of incontinence

Louise ME Wykes

In modern society, an inability to regulate urine output from the body is considered a social disadvantage and will frequently result in the sufferer feeling outcast and ostracised. Their overriding desire may therefore be to maintain secrecy about the problem. Despite the social stigma attached to the condition it is very common, with upwards of three million people in the UK estimated as being incontinent to varying degrees. About half of these are over 65 years of age, and in adults it is a problem that primarily affects women. A willingness by the sufferer to accept that there is a problem, together with an awareness that many others are in a similar situation, may often be a significant psychological advance in the successful management of urinary incontinence.

Once the condition is recognised and accepted, there are many constructive ways in which the general practitioner and pharmacist can assist in its management.

Micturition

A brief description of bladder and allied anatomy and of the normal process of micturition will help in understanding the problems of incontinence. Urine formed in the kidneys passes along the ureters in steady peristaltic waves (occurring about every 10 seconds) and enters the bladder through an opening in its base (Figure 2.1). The bladder is used as a reservoir and as a pump. As a reservoir, it distends as it fills until a sensation is produced which requires it to be emptied. During the process of filling, the bladder is prevented from emptying by the constriction of two sphincters:

- The bladder neck (internal) sphincter, located at the junction of the urethra and bladder
- The external sphincter, located about 3 cm below (i.e nearer the outside) the bladder neck sphincter (also referred to as the voluntary sphincter, as its action may be consciously controlled).

The external sphincter lies within the pelvic floor muscle mass, which also supports the bladder (Figure 2.1). Enhancement of external sphincter action may be achieved by voluntary contraction of this muscle mass.

As a pump, the detrusor muscular wall of the bladder contracts, reducing all the dimensions of the bladder and promoting the evacuation of urine. Controlled emptying occurs through stimulation of the parasympathetic nervous system, which produces contraction of the smooth muscle of bladder wall and relaxation of the internal sphincter. Central nervous control is mediated through these nerves, which arise from the sacral portion of the spinal cord and convey information about the state of the bladder to the brain. Under normal circumstances, an awareness of bladder fullness may occur when about 150 mL of urine has accumulated. Filling usually continues until the volume of urine has risen to about 300 mL.

Bladder control is absent at birth. In the newborn baby, emptying occurs as soon as the bladder is full enough to generate stretching of the muscle fibres, which respond elastically by contracting. Contraction induces a rise in internal pressure, causing urine to be voided. Control of micturition is gradually achieved as the nervous system develops from birth onwards. Most children have daytime control by two years of age. By the time they reach their fourth birthday, most children also remain dry through the night. However, about 10% may still wet the bed at five

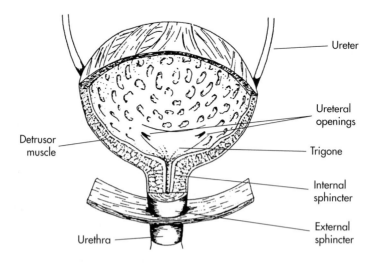

Figure 2.1 Anatomy of the bladder and associated structures.

years of age, and up to 5% may still have occasional bed-wetting episodes even at 10 years of age.

The classification of incontinence

A situation in which normal control of urinary output has been lost and which results in a social or hygiene problem is described as incontinence. A classification of incontinence has been devised based on the clinical history presented by the patient.

Stress incontinence

As the name implies, leakage of urine occurs when any form of physical stress is experienced by the patient. Coughing, sneezing, laughing, exercising, and even just turning over in bed, are activities that may produce a rise in intra-abdominal pressure. Leakage usually occurs because the sphincter mechanisms are weak and failing.

Stress incontinence is the most common form of incontinence, occurring particularly in women after childbirth, when the pelvic floor muscle mass is weakened. Postnatal exercises for the pelvic floor muscles (see below), conscientiously performed, can significantly reduce the incidence of the condition. Stress incontinence may also be aggravated in women postmenopausally, owing to oestrogen deficiencies.

Stress incontinence is rare in men and is usually caused by surgery. It commonly occurs after a prostatectomy. Unlike the other forms of incontinence, stress incontinence usually occurs unexpectedly, with no prior sense of urgency or increased frequency of micturition.

Urge incontinence

Urge incontinence is caused by overactivity of the detrusor muscle in the bladder. A sudden, strong desire to empty the bladder will result in incontinence if the toilet is not reached in time. Urge incontinence is commonly due to the bladder not properly relaxing during filling, or to a loss of central control of bladder contraction (for instance in Parkinson's disease or multiple sclerosis). Frequency of micturition may be increased and incontinence may occur on stress or movement. Gynaecological surgery and drugs (e.g. thiazide and loop diuretics) may also be contributing factors. Other causes include any condition where the lining of the bladder is irritated (e.g. by urinary tract infection). Prostate gland enlargement in men may also produce bladder instability owing to the increased pressure generated around the outlet of the bladder.

Overflow incontinence

Urinary retention may occur if there is urethral obstruction and constriction, or increased intra-abdominal pressure. Prostatic obstruction (e.g. caused by hyperplasia or cancer) and severe constipation are common causes of partial blockage of urinary outflow. Small amounts of urine may then dribble intermittently or continuously from the bladder but, paradoxically, complete voiding may be impossible owing to overdistension of the bladder. It may also occur in women with a large cystocele.

Removal of the central control that causes uninhibited bladder contraction (e.g. after a cerebrovascular incident) gives rise to an effect similar to blocking. Patients suffering from multiple sclerosis or diabetes often also suffer from incontinence that may be classified as overflow or urge incontinence.

Enuresis

Enuresis (bed-wetting) is a form of urge incontinence. Urine leakage occurs because the patient has no sensation of bladder fullness or has an overactive bladder. It most commonly occurs at night (nocturnal enuresis), but daytime enuresis may also occur. The term 'enuresis' is usually taken to apply to children who are wet more than occasionally by day or by night after five years of age.

Enuresis may be a symptom of a more serious disorder, but in most children there may be no emotional or psychiatric disturbances. Conditions associated with enuresis include urinary tract infection, obstructive lesions of the urethra and bladder neck, and neuropathic bladder (e.g. in spina bifida and other spinal disorders). Generalised behavioural disorders may also be a factor in producing bed-wetting. Domestic disharmony or parental disapproval may aggravate the condition.

Miscellaneous causes of incontinence

Emotional stress (as opposed to physical, e.g. before an interview or after bereavement) is a frequent cause of temporary incontinence in adults. 'Accidents' also occur more frequently in the elderly, owing to confusion, reduced mobility and limited manual dexterity. Postmicturition dribble may be a problem, especially for elderly men.

Appliances and their selection

A range of appliances for urinary incontinence is available for both men and women. In England and Wales, items which may be prescribed at NHS expense (on Form FP10) are listed in the *Drug Tariff*, Sections IXA and IXB, and these are specified in Table 2.1. The discussion of how to select an appropriate appliance (see below) is based on the availability of appliances.

There are many aids for incontinence which are not available on Form FP10, although their non-availability from the NHS does not necessarily mean that the patient will have to pay for them. Alternative sources include the community nursing service or school GPs, subject to availability in a particular district. Others may be purchased by the patient from pharmacy stockists or direct from mail-order companies.

In determining the requirements of the incontinent patient, the problem and its causes should be assessed by the doctor or incontinence nurse. The following problems must be considered when selecting an appropriate appliance:

- Is the patient male or female? Most of the satisfactory appliances for the incontinent which may be prescribed are only appropriate for male patients (e.g. drainable dribbling devices and incontinence sheaths). Most of the satisfactory appliances for women, with the exception of catheters, are not prescribable.

Table 2.1 Availability of items for urinary incontinence at NHS expense in England and Wales

Items prescribable	Items not allowed
Urethral catheters	Incontinence pads
Anal plugs	Incontinence garments
Catheter valves	Skin wipes
Drainable dribbling appliances	Occlusive devices (e.g. female vaginal
Faecal collectors	devices and penile clamps)
Incontinence belts	
Incontinence sheaths	
Incontinence sheath fixing strips and adhesives	
Leg bags	
Night drainage bags	
Suspensory systems	
Tubing and accessories	
Urinal systems	

- How severe or regular is the incontinence? The capacity of any urine-collection device must take into consideration the volume and frequency of urine leakage. A patient with only minor dribbling does not require a large-capacity appliance. If the appliance is to be used at night, one with an appropriate capacity must be selected.
- Does the patient possess good manual dexterity and mobility? Patients are less likely to tolerate catheterisation when they are mobile, but this is a particularly useful form of treatment for bedridden patients.

The adhesive properties of materials used to keep appliances in position (e.g. tapes) must be capable of withstanding normal movement to ensure patient confidence in the appliance.

Many appliances require regular emptying, and it is important to ensure that the patient possesses the manual capability to undo drainage points. This may pose an especial problem for elderly patients, who may also be confused about the use of the appliance.

Drainable dribbling devices

The limited capacity of drainable dribbling devices makes them suitable only for men with mild intermittent or continuous dribbling incontinence. This type of incontinence may occur in overflow (see above). Only those appliances that act solely as collection devices are prescribable. Those that contain an absorbent material to soak up urine are not allowed at NHS expense (see Body-worn pants and pads, below).

The device may be held in position by a waist belt with underleg straps, or by drawstrings tied around the scrotum. If the degree of incontinence worsens, dribble collection devices can be linked by a drainage tube connected to a larger collection vessel.

The capacity of most drainable dribbling devices is up to 100 mL, although some may be capable of holding 500 mL. Most devices may be washed and reused for up to a month.

Incontinence sheaths

Incontinence sheaths (penile sheaths, external catheters or condom urinals) are less conspicuous than drainable dribbling devices and may be better tolerated by patients. They may be formed of:

- soft, flexible latex which tapers to a more rigid outlet. Some sheaths incorporate a foam cushion at their base to minimise the risk of abrasion of the end of the penis
- a thicker, less flexible latex into which the outlet tube is moulded.

Both types of sheath are usually available in a range of sizes. Manufacturers may provide guides for measuring the correct size. Diameter or circumference measurements, rather than length, are commonly required for correct fitting. A sheath at least 3 cm longer than the penis should be selected. This prevents irritation of the tip of the penis by the outlet tube and provides spare capacity for sudden spurts of larger volumes of urine.

The outlet from an incontinence sheath must be connected to a drainage bag (which must be separately prescribed) that can be emptied whenever the patient wishes. Most drainage bags are produced with tubing that fits into the outlet of the sheath, although it must be stressed that connections made by different manufacturers are not interchangeable.

The main problem with the use of incontinence sheaths is keeping them in position. Patient confidence in their use may be enhanced by the use of fixative agents. Internal or external adhesive strips can be used to keep the sheath in place. External methods of attachment allow rapid fixation of the sheath. Devices include foam or latex strips held in place by elastic and Velcro fasteners or by adhesives.

Internal methods of fixation (i.e. between the sheath and the skin) tend to produce a more secure bond than external methods. Internal methods range from adhesive coatings placed on the inner surface of the sheath, to separate double-sided adhesive strips made of either foam or a 'stomahesive-type' material which is wrapped around the penis in a spiral. Both are easy to use, as the sheath is usually packed rolled up and unrolls when fitted over the adhesive strip or directly over the skin.

It is essential to ensure that any devices that keep the sheath in position are used carefully. Prolonged constriction of the penis produced by overzealous tightening of the adhesive strip may cause ulceration and, in severe cases, gangrene.

Most incontinence sheaths can be kept in place for up to three days, although it is normally recommended that the device should be changed daily to maintain adequate hygiene of the genitalia.

Leg and night-drainage bags

Leg and night-drainage bags are used to collect urine which drains from urethral catheters or incontinence sheaths. Bags vary considerably in capacity, but the following may be used as general guidelines for their selection:

- Capacity 350–500 mL (small) – for daytime use
- Capacity 750 mL or more (large) – for night-time use.

Most daytime bags for ambulant patients are attached to the leg by straps or supported by a pouch and belt (Figure 2.2). As suspensory systems distribute the weight of urine more evenly, they may be more comfortable than leg straps. The position of the drainage bag on the limb determines the length of the connection tubing from the catheter or sheath (where there is a choice). The length of the inlet tube corresponds to the position on the leg as follows:

- Thigh position – about 5 cm
- Knee position – 10 cm
- Calf – >10 cm.

Bags are attached by straps manufactured in a range of materials (e.g. latex, foam and Velcro, or elastic). Leg straps for use by women should be selected so as not to damage clothing (e.g. hosiery).

Drainage bags may be constructed of plastic or rubber. Those made of plastic have a life of five to seven days. Rubber bags are less commonly used, although they may last four to six months with careful washing between uses. However, continued reuse may lead to the development of odour and an increased risk of urinary tract infection. If the urine is already infected, absorbed ammoniacal odours may be impossible to eradicate completely. As plastic surfaces can cause discomfort when worn next to the skin, some drainage bags have a woven backing.

The choice of a drainage bag may be governed in part by the design of its outlet tap. The patient must be capable of manually removing and replacing the outlet tap, or carrying out whatever procedure is required for drainage. Removable caps (which may be easily dropped or mislaid) and those with special mechanisms may pose problems for some patients (especially the elderly and the confused).

Many collection devices incorporate a non-return valve at the connection point of the tubing from the catheter or sheath and the inlet port. This is particularly useful for bedridden patients, whose bag and tubing may inadvertently lie in the same horizontal plane as the patient. The non-return valve may also reduce the risk of ascending bacterial infection.

When the bag has to rest on the floor, hangers may be available from the community nursing service, although they are not prescribable.

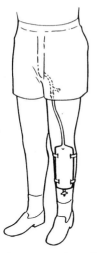

Leg bag strapped to calf

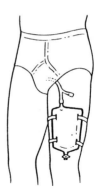

Leg bag strapped to thigh

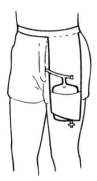

Leg bag with holster

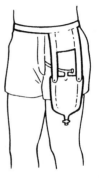

Leg bag with sporan

Figure 2.2 Drainage bag support systems.

Body-worn urinal systems

Body-worn urinal systems are specialised devices comprising a number of parts. One disadvantage of their use is the difficulty an untrained person may experience in assembling and fitting the system. Patients prescribed such systems should possess good mental capacity and manual dexterity, or be in the care of someone who can carry out correct assembly, fitting and maintenance.

The main parts of a urinal comprise:

- a channelling device (e.g. cone or sheath) which is held in position by a waist band and understraps
- a collection device (e.g. bag) which may be held to the leg by straps or left unattached.

Differences between urinals arise in the design of the channelling device. The five main types are described below.

Pubic pressure urinal

The penis is inserted through a plate which is securely held to the pubis by a waistband and leg understraps (Figure 2.3). When correctly fitted, the pubic pressure urinal may be particularly suited for a patient with a retracted penis. A sheath is attached to the pubic plate. If the patient is confined to bed, an internal sheath may help to prevent backflow of urine around and under the plate.

Diaphragm-type urinal

The plate and sheath of a pubic pressure urinal are replaced by a single diaphragm through which the penis is inserted. Scrotal supports can also be added.

Sheath-type urinal

A detachable sheath fits inside a cone which channels urine into a collection bag. The cone is less rigid than in a pubic pressure urinal and can be more easily dislodged.

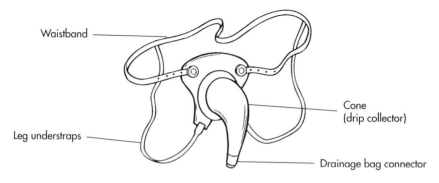

Figure 2.3 Pubic pressure urinal.

Penile and scrotal-type urinal

If the penis is too small to allow satisfactory attachment of the urinals described above, an alternative device is available which encloses the penis and scrotum within a sac.

Drip-type urinal

Unlike the other urinals described here, a drip-type urinal does not have a collection bag attached to it. It is intended for use in overflow incontinence in which a small volume (50–100 mL) of urine may collect in the sheath. The urine is drained through a replaceable screw-cap outlet. Most devices can be converted to night-time use by attachment of a drainage bag and connecting tube.

Ordering information

The following must be specified when complete urinals are ordered:

- Penile circumference, measured adjacent to the surface of the skin. If the urinal is one-size only, there is usually an internal sheath that must be cut to size
- Waist measurement, which is often defined as 'standard', although outsize patients may require special fittings.

Most patients require two complete urinal sets, one being in use while the other is washed on alternate days in mild soap and water. Each urinal should be immersed weekly in an antiseptic fluid. With proper care and cleansing, each appliance should last for six months.

Many urinal components may be ordered separately. For full details, consult the manufacturer.

Female body-worn urinals

Because of the obvious anatomical differences, body-worn urinals for women are far less satisfactory than those described above for men.

The channelling component of the female urinal is positioned between the legs and held in place by waist-belt loops. To improve comfort, devices may have an inflatable cuff around the urinal opening. Urine which enters the urinal is collected in a drainable bag attached to the leg.

Urethral catheters

Catheterisation has been used in many different forms for thousands of years, although it is only in recent years that its use has been relatively successful. In some respects, the use of a catheter reflects a failure to manage a patient's incontinence by other, less invasive means. However, in many cases, and in women in particular, catheterisation is one of the few satisfactory methods of treatment.

For the chronically incontinent patient, each catheter is left in position for as long as possible (an indwelling catheter). Conversely, short-term catheterisation may be used postoperatively. Although most long-term catheterisation is continuous, there is an increasing trend towards the use of intermittent catheterisation, particularly in spina bifida and spinal injury patients. One advantage of intermittent catheterisation is the preservation of the patient's dignity.

Indwelling catheters are connected to a drainage bag which holds the urine. The bag is emptied as required through a tap. Alternatively, there may be a catheter valve which is released at regular intervals.

Catheters may be classified as Nelaton, Scott or Foley types. The Nelaton catheter consists of a long, continuous tube with eyes at the end inserted into the bladder, and a connecting attachment at the opposite end (Figure 2.4a). Nelaton catheters may be used for intermittent catheterisation. The catheter is inserted every two to four hours, or as instructed by the clinician.

The Scott catheter is made of slightly more rigid plastic and is specifically for female use (Figure 2.4b). It is used for intermittent catheterisation and may only be supplied on FP10NC and FP10C when specifically ordered.

The Foley catheter incorporates a side arm through which sterile water can be introduced (Figure 2.4c). Once the catheter has been inserted into the bladder, sterile water is passed along a channel to inflate a balloon near the tip of the catheter; the balloon then acts as a self-retaining device.

Balloon size

The self-retaining devices have varying capacities when inflated:

- 5 mL – for paediatric use
- 10 mL, 20 mL and 30 mL – for adult use.

If the balloon size is not specified, the 10 mL size should be supplied. The 10 mL balloon has the advantage of being smaller and causing less

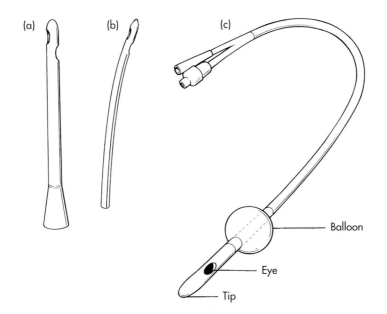

(a) (b) (c)

Balloon

Eye

Tip

Figure 2.4 Types of catheter. (a) Nelaton catheter, (b) Scott catheter, (c) Foley catheter.

downward pressure on the trigone muscle. In addition, the eyes of the catheter sit lower in the bladder, so reducing the volume of pooled, stagnant urine at the base of the bladder. However, the catheter with a 10 mL balloon can be more easily pulled out, especially by confused or demented patients.

The 30 mL balloon is for patients whose bladder neck muscles are particularly weak (e.g. after prostatectomy).

Material of construction

The choice of construction material for a catheter depends on the expected duration of catheterisation.

Catheters made of latex are the cheapest but most seldom used. They are recommended for short-term catheterisation only. The pitted, molecular structure of the latex produces encrustation after only a couple of days, and the internal channel is quickly blocked. In practice, one catheter generally lasts one to two weeks. Latex may be coated with a low-resistance material (e.g. Teflon or silicone). The coating reduces the roughness of the latex surface, but its presence effectively reduces the internal diameter of the channel. Teflon-coated latex catheters are for short-term catheterisation. Silicone-coated catheters are for medium–long-term catheterisation.

Plastic-PVC is used for intermittent-use catheters. It resists encrustation longer than latex (up to two weeks) and is used especially post-operatively, when the urine contains a lot of debris. However, these catheters can be uncomfortable because of their rigidity, and care must be taken on insertion not to damage bladder or urethral tissue.

All-silicone catheters are the products of choice for long-term catheterisation. Because of a different method of manufacture, the internal diameter of an all-silicone catheter is much greater than that of one made from latex. As a result, drainage rates are improved and the rate of encrustation is reduced. Silicone also provokes a lesser immune reaction than latex and may be associated with a reduced risk of urinary tract infection. The all-silicone catheter can remain in place for up to 12 weeks, although the balloon may deflate and requires periodic checking.

Hydrogel-coated catheters are for long-term catheterisation. The coating reduces friction on insertion and resists encrustation. The catheter can last up to 12 weeks and fewer problems are encountered during use than with other catheter materials.

Catheter gauge

The Charrière (Ch) system or French gauge (FG) (with even numbers only) is used to define the external catheter diameter in millimetres, and therefore reflects the internal channel diameter. The 14 Ch to 24 Ch sizes can be recognised by the internationally accepted colour codes on the inflation arm (Table 2.2). Where no gauge is specified, size 14 Ch or 16 Ch should be supplied.

Paediatric catheters are usually size 6–10 Ch. For most adult users, sizes 14–16 Ch are appropriate. Larger gauges should only be used when there is considerable debris (e.g. from blood clots after surgery, or from mucus). Use of a large-diameter catheter may aggravate these states through irritation and further damage to the bladder wall.

Catheter length

The different lengths of catheters used by men and women reflect the differences in anatomy. Catheters for adult males are about 40 cm in length. Catheters for adult females range from 18 to 26 cm. Paediatric devices for males are about 30 cm in length.

Table 2.2 Foley catheters

Charrière size (French gauge)	Approximate external diameter (mm)	International colour code
6	2.00	–
8	2.66	–
10	3.33	–
12	4.00	–
14	4.66	Green
16	5.33	Brown/orange
18	6.00	Red
20	6.66	Yellow
22	7.33	Violet/purple
24	8.00	Blue
26	8.66	–
28	9.33	–
30	10.00	–

Problems with catheter use

One of the main reasons why long-term catheterisation should always be considered a last resort in the management of incontinence is that urinary tract infection is invariably a consequence. Infection ascending to the kidneys produces renal damage and accounts for 20–40% of all deaths of catheterised patients.

The risk of introducing infection is considerably increased on each occasion that the connection between the catheter and collection device is broken, and by frequent, unnecessary catheter changing. The use of modern technology to produce smooth uncracked surfaces greatly reduces the development of blockage and encrustation, and has allowed the period between catheter changes to increase. In addition, the greater internal diameter of all-silicone catheters (compared to latex or silicone-coated latex materials) allows the use of smaller gauge sizes. As a result, a smaller 'immune' response from the body to the foreign material may be provoked, with less debris and fewer white blood cells generated.

Previously, regular twice-weekly irrigation of the bladder through the catheter was practised, using chlorhexidine or saline. This was done in the belief that the incidence of infection and catheter obstruction would be reduced. This is no longer recommended, as an increased, rather than decreased, risk of infection has now been identified.

When urinary tract infection is present, the use of a newly de-veloped, easier-to-use bladder washout system has been shown to be effective. Systems containing antiseptics (e.g. chlorhexidine), agents for dissolving internal catheter encrustation (e.g. citric acid) or catheter-flushing agents (e.g. normal saline) are available for catheter care.

Handheld urinals (male and female)

In conjunction with specially adapted clothing (e.g. wraparound skirts), handheld urinals are a useful aid in the management of incontinence, particularly for those patients who are unable to reach a toilet quickly.

The choice of urinal depends on a number of factors. With some urinals, the patient must be physically capable of lifting themselves on to or over the device; this may be impossible for those who are weak or immobile. Manual dexterity and strength must also be assessed if urinals with or without handles are to be used.

Spillage during and after use is an especial problem. Male urinals may incorporate a non-return valve to minimise this risk (Figure 2.5a). Others include a cap which can be easily snapped on after the urinal has been used (Figure 2.5b). Spillage may be a more significant problem with female urinals because of the requirement for a wider opening. The use of a waterproof PVC sheet between the user and clothing or bedding may be a useful measure for a patient with a high risk of spillage.

Female urinals are positioned between the legs from the front, or are straddled or sat on. The bridge urinal (Figure 2.6a) may be used

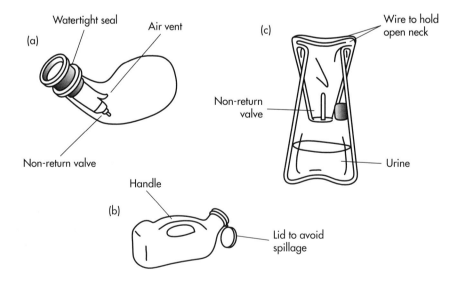

Figure 2.5 Handheld male urinals.

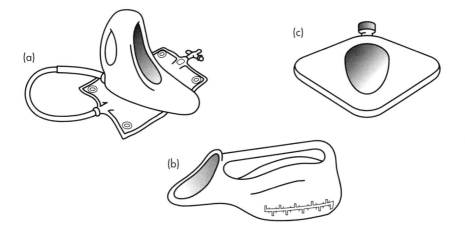

Figure 2.6 Handheld female urinals. (a) Bridge urinal, (b) cygnet urinal, (c) triangular urinal.

alone or may be attached to a drainage bag. It is preferred by the immobile, as it can be attached to a wheelchair and removes the need to raise the body. The cygnet urinal (Figure 2.6b) is bottle-shaped and may be used when standing, sitting, or lying on the side. The triangular urinal (Figure 2.6c) is shallow and may be used when sitting.

Most urinals are made of rigid plastic and should be cleaned daily after use by rinsing with a disinfectant solution or soaking in warm, soapy water. Cleaning may be done with warm water and a chlorhexidine solution. Sodium hypochlorite solutions may be effective in cleaning plastic appliances but are harmful to rubber-based materials. Chloroxylenol may be a suitable alternative for appliances containing rubber. Disposable, more flexible, plastic urinals are also available and are in effect plastic bags supported on a rigid plastic frame (Figure 2.5c). They are expensive for routine use, but may be a suitable alternative to the rigid type where cleaning facilities are less readily available (e.g. on holiday).

Body-worn pads and pants

In patients with infrequent mild incontinence, pads and pants may provide the necessary degree of protection and at the same time give patients the confidence to lead a full and normal life. A wide variety of products are available, including both pads worn under ordinary clothes and special absorbent pads. In each case the products may be disposable or washable.

Pads

Disposable pads are most commonly used to manage incontinence. They are held in place by close-fitting pants, stretch pants or pants with a pouch. The insert pads may be shaped, elasticated, or have adhesive strips, and many different sizes and absorbencies are available. Pads containing superabsorbers, which are able to absorb 50 times their own weight, have recently been developed. Wetness indicators and waterproof backing are features also incorporated in some pads.

Male pouches are suitable for men with slight or dribbling incontinence (Figure 2.7a). These have an adhesive strip to keep them in position and may be worn with close-fitting pants.

All-in-one disposables have elasticated legs and resealable side tapes. They are suitable for heavy urinary or faecal incontinence and may be favoured by those confined to bed or a wheelchair. All-in-one washable garments are fastened by press studs or Velcro, and are generally more secure than the adhesive tabs of the disposable products.

Pants

Absorbent washable pants have a waterproof-backed pad sewn into them. Most are only suitable for slight urinary incontinence, although some can handle moderate to severe incontinence. The advantages of these are that they look like ordinary pants and the pads cannot be removed inappropriately. However, every pad change means a change of underwear, which may be inconvenient.

Pouch pants are suitable for a light to moderate amount of urine, but not for faecal incontinence. The pad is worn in the pouch (Figure 2.7b), leaving a layer of fabric between the skin and the pad. The fabric is hydrophobic, which means the surface in contact with the skin remains dry. Pads may be changed when necessary, but some designs require considerable manual dexterity.

Drop-front pants enable the pad to be removed without the need for the pants to be taken down. The drop-front flap may be fastened with Velcro or studs, which can be easily undone and refastened. Bikini-type pants tied at each side of the waist are available as an alternative to drop-front pants.

Most pants can be ordered according to the waist size of the patient and/or the capacity of the pad.

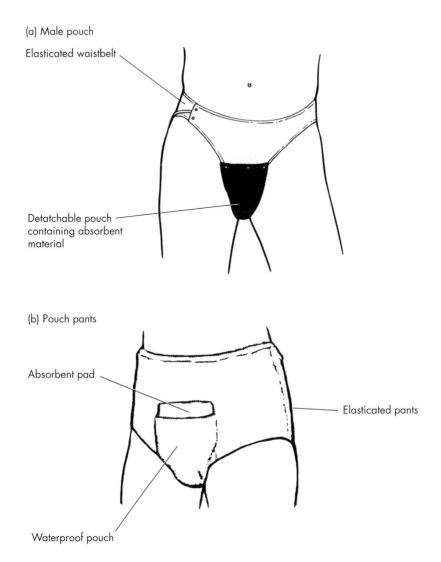

(a) Male pouch

Elasticated waistbelt

Detatchable pouch
containing absorbent
material

(b) Pouch pants

Absorbent pad

Elasticated pants

Waterproof pouch

Figure 2.7 Absorbent pouches. (a) Male pouch, (b) pouch pants.

Anal plug

This is a small foam tampon which is inserted into the anus, where it expands. It can be left in place for 12 hours, although it will need to be removed for a bowel movement.

Other aids to continence

Bed and chair pads (i.e. not body worn) consist of cellulose wadding with a plastic backing and are placed between the patient and the furniture. They are not very satisfactory as a means of management and their use implies that there is no other protection (which may be necessary), or that the primary form of protection has failed.

Mattress and bedding protection may be used to allow the patient to obtain an undisturbed night's sleep, particularly if infrequent episodes of incontinence do not warrant more permanent aids.

Odour control, particularly after incontinence has occurred, may be an important factor in allowing patients to regain confidence and resume normal activities. However, the smell produced by a deodorant should not be recognisable as one associated with the leakage of urine or the presence of stale urine.

Exercising pelvic floor muscles

The importance of the integrity of the external bladder sphincter in maintaining urinary continence has already been emphasised (see above). Contraction of the pelvic floor muscles controls the ability to stop voiding urine in mid stream. During pregnancy and childbirth these muscles may be severely stretched. Exercises can help to strengthen them and prevent the development, or reduce the occurrence, of stress incontinence.

Exercises should be done for a minimum of seven to eight weeks, and ideally for up to six months. The guidelines below should be followed:

- Patients should initially be taught to consciously tighten and relax the muscles around the anus while standing, sitting or lying down.
- Patients should then be asked to sit on the toilet or commode and start to pass urine. In mid stream they should try to stop the flow by contracting the urethral muscles. Once this has been done satisfactorily, they ought to be aware of the different sets of muscles that control the anus and the urethra.
- The exercises can then be done sitting, standing or lying down. Patients must make a conscious effort to contract the anal and urethral muscles, initially alternately and subsequently in unison. On contraction, the muscle should be held for approximately four seconds and then released. The exercise should be repeated up to four times each hour, and may be done at any convenient time.

A number of intravaginal devices are available to help with pelvic floor exercises. These include vaginal cones, which are weighted, requiring the pelvic floor muscles to be contracted to keep the cone inside the vagina. Other devices (e.g. Contiform and the Conveen continence guard) are designed to give support to the bladder neck. A battery-operated unit may also be used to contract the pelvic floor muscles by applying electrical stimulation via a vaginal electrode. These devices cannot be prescribed at NHS expense (Table 2.1).

Enuresis alarms

In children with persistent enuresis (bed-wetting) a considerable emotional and physical strain may be placed on the child and the family. Support from community services (i.e. the GP and allied healthcare professionals) may provide the reassurance and assistance necessary to break the 'habit' of recurrent episodes. Other external devices may also aid in management of the condition.

Enuresis alarms consist of a sensor pad which detects urine. The pad is linked to a control unit, which provides an auditory, vibratory or visual stimulus (i.e. bell, buzzer or light) that is intended to wake the child before complete voiding occurs.

The sensor device may consist of two sheets of wire mesh or perforated metal foil separated by a thin cloth. The sensor pad is placed under the lower bedsheet, and the presence of urine completes the electrical circuit by bridging the space between the two metal sheets. When the child is woken by the alarm they get out of bed, switch off the alarm, empty their bladder, and reset the alarm under a dry sheet before returning to bed. One drawback of this method is that the child may sleep through the alarm, or reset it semiconsciously without voiding urine. One way to overcome this is to place the alarm far enough from the bed to make the child get up to switch it off.

The 'Nottingham' alarm may also be used, in which a sensor probe is inserted into a sanitary pad worn by the child inside a pair of underpants. The alarm is wired into a small box which may be pinned to the child's nightclothes. The device may also be used during the day.

Useful addresses

In addition to the doctor, the district (or home) nurse and the health visitor may be able to advise the patient on the supply of personal equipment for the management of incontinence. The nurse or health visitor may be able to help the patient to take advantage of a laundry service and a collection service for the disposal of soiled pads and other disposable items.

The social worker and occupational therapist may be able to provide information on the availability of home helps, grants for alterations to toilet and bathroom facilities in the home, and the supply of commodes and chemical closets.

Age Concern England
Astral House
1268 London Road
London SW16 4ER
Tel: 0800 009966
www.ageconcern.org.uk

Association for Continence Advice
102a Astra House
Arklow Road
New Cross
London SE14 6EB
Tel: 020 8692 4680
www.aca.uk.com/mainindex.html

Enuresis Resource and Information Centre (ERIC)
34 Old School House
Britannia Road
Kingswood
Bristol BS15 8DB
Tel: 0117 9603060
www.eric.org.uk

Help The Aged
St James's Walk
Clerkenwell Green
London EC1R 0BE
Tel: 020 7253 0253
www.helptheaged.org.uk

Incontact
Freepost Lon 12119
London SE1 1BT
Tel: 020 7717 1225

Promocon 2001
Redbank House
St Chad's Street
Cheetham
Manchester M8 8QA
Tel: 0161 834 2001
e-mail: promocon2001@disabledliving.co.uk

The Continence Foundation
307 Hatton Square
16 Baldwins Gardens
London EC1N 7RJ
Tel: 020 7831 9831
www.continence-foundation.org.uk

3

Trusses for abdominal hernias

Louise ME Wykes

A hernia or rupture is a protrusion of the bowel through a weakened part of (usually) the abdominal muscle wall. This weakening often develops over a period of time, but the hernia may arise suddenly as a result of a bout of coughing, lifting heavy weights, or doing heavy manual work. Straining at stool because of constipation may also be a factor. The abdominal muscle mass has several potential weak points where a hernia may develop.

Types of hernia

Inguinal hernia

The most common kind of hernia is an inguinal hernia, in which weakness occurs in the inguinal canal located either side of the lower abdomen just above the groin. In an indirect inguinal hernia the hernial sac passes through the inguinal canal. In a direct inguinal hernia the hernial sac pushes through the muscular wall of the abdomen to protrude at the external opening of the inguinal canal.

An inguinal hernia usually increases in size the further down the inguinal canal it occurs. If it is below the pubic arch it is termed a scrotal hernia.

Umbilical hernia

The umbilicus is an area of potential weakness, and an umbilical hernia is particularly common in overweight adults and in women during or after pregnancy. It also occurs in infants through the umbilical scar.

Femoral hernia

A femoral hernia is less common than other types of hernia and its incidence is greater in women. The protrusion is found at the top of the thigh, just below the groin adjacent to the femoral artery. Femoral hernias are particularly prone to strangulation (see below).

Other hernias

In addition to the sites illustrated in Figure 3.1, any abdominal operation scar represents potential weakening in the muscle mass, and the pressure of abdominal contents at such points may develop into a hernia.

Management of hernias

A hernia may be corrected surgically, and in some instances this is an urgent requirement, particularly where there is a risk of strangulation (see below). However, a mechanical means of support (a truss) may be necessary:

- in the interval between diagnosis and surgical correction
- because the patient is too old or too ill to withstand surgery.

The use of a truss for hernial support may therefore be a temporary or a long-term measure.

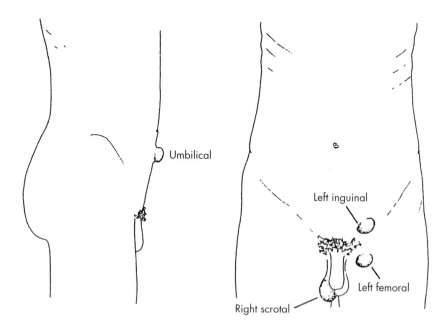

Figure 3.1 Positions of hernias.

'Reducing' a hernia

Before an appliance can be used for hernial support, it must be demonstrated that the protruding abdominal mass can be returned through the weakened muscle into the abdominal cavity. This process is known as 'reducing' the hernia, and such a hernia is said to be 'reducible'. Because of the significant risk of strangulation (see below), a truss must not be supplied or fitted to a hernia that will not reduce. Occasionally, reduction may be achieved simply by getting the patient to lie down, particularly when the hernial mass is small and relatively firm. If lying down does not reduce the hernia, manipulating it in an upward direction with one hand and in a backward direction with the other will usually return the mass to the abdominal cavity. The hernia should not be forced. Raising the knee on the same side of the body as the hernia and inclining the body to the opposite side may aid reduction. It must also be demonstrated that the patient can successfully reduce the hernia themself.

If the hernia is small and not readily visible, its position can be confirmed by palpation. The doctor, pharmacist or nurse should place their fingers over the approximate site of the hernia and the patient should be asked to cough. An outward thrusting force can then be felt at the point of weakness.

Strangulation of a hernia

A hernia is said to be 'strangulated' if its blood supply is cut off. Strangulation is a serious condition requiring immediate medical attention.

Selection of the correct truss

A truss consists of a pad which is placed over the reduced hernia. The pad is kept in place by a belt, which may be made of a rigid spring or flexible elastic. The belt also helps the pad to exert an upward and backward force.

The pad

Pads are individually shaped for the different types of hernia described above, and each design is available in a range of sizes.

Inguinal hernia pads

These are oval in shape. The main body of the pad is placed over the site of the hernia.

Scrotal hernia pads

These have an elongated lower portion which supports the lower end of the inguinal canal below the pubic arch. The elongated portion may often be referred to as a 'rat-tail', as the end of the pad continues between the thighs and round to the rear of the waist support.

Femoral hernia pads

These incorporate many of the characteristics of both inguinal and scrotal pads. The femoral pad is more difficult to keep in position than either the inguinal or the scrotal pad, as it lies at the top of the thigh.

Umbilical hernia pads

For adults these consist of a padded plate with a central raised cone. The cone, which is held in position by the plate, sits over the umbilicus. An umbilical hernia in a child is usually very small and is commonly caused by excessive crying. An appropriate device for children is a porous indiarubber belt which, unlike the adult version, does not have a central cone. An elastic webbing belt (which is not prescribable) may be preferred if the patient is sensitive to rubber.

The belt

Elastic band

The elastic band truss is more popular with the wearer than the spring truss as it is less obtrusive below clothing and feels more comfortable. This may be especially important for a patient who has a night-time cough. However, the truss will not stay in place automatically, and the understrap which passes between the thighs is an essential requirement. The elastic band truss also decreases in effectiveness more rapidly than the spring truss, commonly requiring replacement in less than 12 months.

Spring

As a general rule, a spring truss gives better support to the hernia pad than an elastic belt and is therefore more effective. The force it generates is in direct opposition to the outward tendency of the hernia, whereas that generated by the elastic band is only an indirect force. The pad on a spring truss may stay in place automatically, with only the scrotal version requiring an understrap. A spring truss will lose its tension only slowly if it is put on correctly, and it can provide adequate support for 18 months if properly looked after.

Elastic band and spring trusses are illustrated in Figures 3.2 and 3.3.

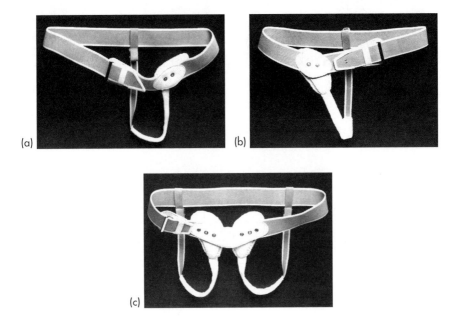

Figure 3.2 Elastic band trusses. (a) Single inguinal, (b) single scrotal, (c) double scrotal.

Measuring for a truss

Correct measurements next to the skin must be taken in order for a satisfactory truss to be supplied.

The measuring tape must be carefully positioned. For inguinal and femoral hernias, the tape placed around the body should lie just above the buttocks at the rear and between the iliac crests (the top edge of the hip bones) and the greater trochanters (hip joints) at each side (Figure 3.4). The actual measurement required for truss fitting should be taken where the tape crosses at the pubis. For umbilical hernias the circumference of the body should be measured at the level of the hernia. In neither case should the actual hernia be measured.

Minor modifications to some adult measurements for spring trusses may be necessary. If the patient is particularly overweight, the tape should

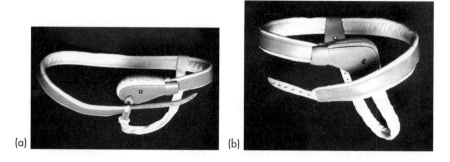

Figure 3.3 Spring trusses. (a) Single inguinal, (b) single scrotal.

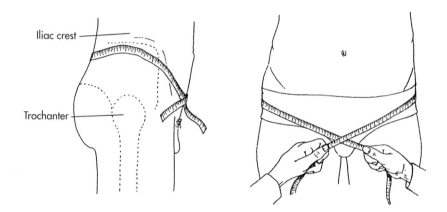

Figure 3.4 Measuring for a truss.

be pulled very tight to ensure that the truss belt is not too big. Conversely, for thin, bony patients slight overmeasurements should be taken to prevent abrasion of the skin over spinal and pelvic bony protrusions.

Fitting the truss

Under the NHS contract, a pharmacist or other trained member of staff must fit a truss when a prescription is presented. Immediatly prior to this, the hernia *must* be reduced with the patient lying down.

An elastic band truss can be placed directly around the waist, with the pad positioned over the reduced hernia. The body band should then be tightened with the patient standing, and the understraps should be fixed to the band at each side, not at the back. A spring truss requires more dexterity and manipulation for correct fitting. It must not be forced open, as this will severely reduce the effectiveness and lifespan of the spring. The truss should be passed around the knees and slid upwards over the buttocks to sit just below the iliac crests.

Correct fitting of the truss may be confirmed by asking the patient to cough. The hernia should be retained under the pad if it is correctly positioned.

Prescribing and ordering information

The following information must be given to ensure the correct supply of a truss:

- Type of pad – inguinal/scrotal/femoral/umbilical
- Size of pad – standard (fitted unless specified)/large/small
- Type of belt – spring/elastic band
- Number of pads – single/double
- Position of pads – right/left/both
- Body circumference measurement – see Measuring for a truss, above.

Items allowed on forms FP10 (as listed in *Drug Tariff* Part IXA) are shown in Tables 3.1 and 3.2.

Table 3.1 Spring trusses allowed on Forms FP10 (*Drug Tariff* Specification 31a)

- Inguinal
- Inguinal rat-tail
- Femoral
- Scrotal
- Double inguinal/scrotal
- Double inguinal/scrotal with extras (back pad, fixed or sliding; slotted, polished spring ends) if ordered
- 'Special' truss with unusually shaped pads (should be confirmed by prescriber)
- Replacements and repairs of understraps for inguinal or femoral trusses

Table 3.2 Elastic band trusses allowed on Forms FP10 (*Drug Tariff* Specification 31b)

- Inguinal
- Scrotal
- Umbilical, single belt
- Umbilical double belt, where specified by prescriber
- 'Special' truss with unusually shaped pads (should be confirmed by prescriber)

Cleaning the pad(s) and belt

It is important to clean the truss correctly to ensure its maximum life. The pad should be lightly sponged, not completely soaked. Elasticated belts may be similarly treated. A spring truss should be wiped over with a damp (not wet) cloth. If the truss is made too wet, the metal inside will rust.

Further reading

Bellingham, C (2002). Successful truss fitting. *Pharm J* 268: 61–62.
The NPA Guide to the Drug Tariff and NHS Dispensing for England and Wales (1999). St Albans: National Pharmaceutical Association, 126–131.

4

Graduated compression hosiery

Louise Whitley

Graduated compression hosiery is used to provide compression and support in conditions related to venous insufficiency or oedema. Graduated compression garments exert the greatest degree of compression at the ankle, and the level of compression gradually decreases up the garment.

Support hosiery is used to prevent the development of leg circulatory problems and to reduce the incidence of tired, aching legs. Support hosiery usually exerts considerably less compression than graduated compression hosiery, and the degree of compression is the same along the length of the garment.

Graduated compression hosiery may be supplied on NHS prescription if it conforms to *Drug Tariff* specifications (see *Drug Tariff*, Appliances Part IXA). Graduated compression hosiery may be prescribed by doctors on form FP10, or by nurses on form FP10(CN) or FP10(PN). Support hosiery is not available at NHS expense.

Indications for graduated compression hosiery

Varicose veins

Graduated compression hosiery is used in the management of varicose veins, venous leg ulcers, post-operative deep vein thrombosis, and oedema. One indication for the use of compression hosiery is varicose veins. These irregular bulbous protrusions may occur in the oesophagus and rectum, but are commonest in the legs. Up to 20% of the population may suffer from varicosities to different degrees, with women being five times as likely as men to develop symptoms.

The causes, prevention and treatment of varicose veins may be best understood through a knowledge of the venous system in the legs.

Relevant physiology

When a person is standing, the flow of venous blood returning to the heart from the lower limbs must take place against gravity. Blood flows from the surface tissue capillaries to the short and long saphenous veins, which lie outside the main muscle mass of the leg (Figure 4.1). The long saphenous vein ascends on the inside of the leg; the short saphenous vein drains blood from the outside areas of the leg. The veins pass through the fibrous sheath which encases the muscle mass of the leg. The long saphenous vein penetrates the muscle sheath near the groin, and the short saphenous vein penetrates the sheath behind the knee. As these

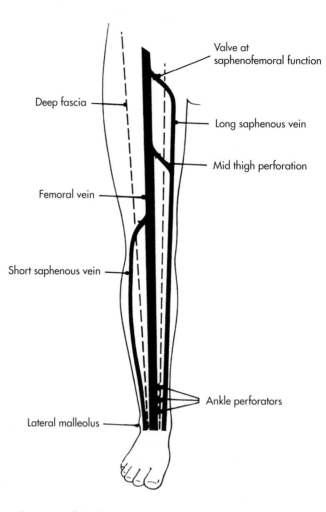

Figure 4.1 The veins of the leg.

veins lie outside the main muscle mass of the leg, the walls of the saphenous veins contain a greater proportion of muscle than other veins of comparable diameter.

The inward and upward movement of the blood continues via communicating or perforator veins to the deep veins that lie within the leg muscle. The small perforator veins, which link the saphenous veins with the deep veins, contain a non-return valve at the point where they penetrate the muscular fibrous sheath (see below). The unidirectional flow of blood is aided by a number of factors:

- Bicuspid valves, which occur at intervals along the veins
- The residual pressure in the venous system from the heart contraction (normally about 16 mmHg), which exerts a mild upward force
- The blood within the deep veins is propelled along by contractions of the leg muscle (the calf muscle pump)
- The pressure within the thorax is less than that in the external environment. A partial 'suction' effect therefore acts to draw blood up from the legs. The increased abdominal pressure that occurs during pregnancy reduces this effect, predisposing expectant women to the development of varicosities.

Varicose veins may develop as a result of detrimental effects on one or more of the above factors. Other positively identified contributory factors are described below.

Contributory factors

Genetics   There is often a well-defined family history of varicose veins. Genetic disposition may even lead to the occurrence of varicosities in identical positions on the legs of a mother and her offspring. This may be partially explained by the observation that the distribution and number of the valves in leg veins may be genetically determined.

Hormones   Oestrogens and progestogens exert a relaxant effect on smooth muscle. The relatively high proportion of smooth muscle in the walls of the saphenous veins predisposes them to hormonal relaxation and therefore increases the susceptibility to pooling of blood and valvular damage. The importance of hormonal influences on the occurrence of varicose veins is further highlighted by the cyclical development of symptoms in many women. In addition, women are up to five times more likely to develop the condition than are men, and painful symptoms are restricted almost entirely to women.

Pregnancy Hormonal changes in early pregnancy and the pressure of the baby on the pelvic veins in the later stages may cause varicose veins. After delivery most varicosities disappear spontaneously, although the mother may be predisposed to redevelop the condition in later life.

Deep vein thrombosis Thrombotic episodes produce obstructions in the deep veins of the leg. The valves in the deep veins are frequently involved and may become ineffective through fibrosis. As a result, blood develops retrograde flow through the deep veins, increasing the pressure on and reducing the competency of valves in the perforating and superficial veins. Pooling of the blood occurs, producing the characteristic varicosities.

Posture Prolonged standing (e.g. at work) may accelerate the development of varicosities. Lack of movement when standing leads to prolonged, unvaried pressure exerted by the leg muscles on the deep veins. This increases the resistance to the return of blood through the venous system and exerts increased pressure on the valves of the perforating and superficial veins.

Abdominal masses The presence of a large bulk within the abdomen over a long period of time can generate pressure changes within the venous system. Abdominal tumours may be a precipitating factor, and it has also been suggested that chronic constipation or obesity may predispose susceptible individuals to the development of varicose veins.

Symptoms

Varicose veins may be associated with aching, fatigue, and a feeling of warmth in the affected veins. Symptoms do not correlate well with the severity of the varicosity: patients with mild varicose veins may experience severe pain, whereas those with severe leg involvement may be asymptomatic. Elevating the leg relieves symptoms. Many patients are concerned by the appearance of varicose veins and find them cosmetically unacceptable.

Complications may occur. These include eczema or changes in the colour of the skin. If there is incompetence of the deep veins, oedema may occur. Ulceration may also develop. Ulcers caused by varicose veins tend to be small, superficial, and extremely painful; those due to deep vein incompetence are usually larger.

Treatment options

Pharmacists are concerned primarily with the use of graduated compression hosiery to alleviate varicose symptoms, but a brief account of other treatment methods is also relevant.

Varicose veins may be treated in one of three ways, although physical compression is invariably a component of compression sclerotherapy and surgery:

- Compression sclerotherapy
- Surgery
- Physical compression.

Compression sclerotherapy   In varicose veins, retrograde flow of venous blood through damaged valves (usually in the perforating veins) leads to pooling of blood in the superficial system. The aim of sclerotherapy is to shut off these damaged channels by local injection of an irritant material into an emptied vein. The irritant damages the inner wall of the vein and produces a microscopic clot. The two walls of the vein are clamped firmly together with a crepe bandage, which should ideally remain in place for four to six weeks. Graduated compression hosiery can be used over the bandage to help to keep it in place and to apply consistent pressure to the whole limb. It may also help prevent recurrence.

Walking is an essential part of postoperative care, and patients who are unable or unwilling to exercise fully after sclerotherapy (e.g. by walking on average four miles a day) are often deemed unsuitable for this treatment. Despite the relative ease of treatment (which may be done on an outpatient basis), the procedure is unsuccessful in 30% of patients.

Surgery   Surgery may be indicated if varicosities are extensive or sclerotherapy has proved unsuccessful. If the superficial veins are grossly dilated, surgery may be carried out. The most commonly used surgical procedures are ligation and stripping.

After surgery, the limb is dressed and firmly bandaged. It is recommended that walking should be resumed as soon as possible after surgery, and that the bandaging is left undisturbed for up to five days. Bandaging may be required for a subsequent period of 10–14 days.

There is a relapse rate of about 20% with this form of treatment. This may be partially attributed to the increased stress to which the remaining veins are subjected as the venous blood finds alternative routes back to the heart. The use of graduated compression hosiery postoperatively can significantly reduce the recurrence of varicose veins.

Physical compression The use of physical compression is a conservative measure which in no way cures varicose veins but aims to prevent their deterioration. However, in view of the relapse rate for sclerotherapy and surgery, the use of compression alone may be considered acceptable in many cases. This is particularly so in the early stages of the condition, in pregnancy, and also where the above techniques are contraindicated (e.g. in immobile or incapacitated patients).

Compression is beneficial to a patient with reduced venous function for a variety of reasons. Distension of the superficial veins caused by the presence of high internal pressure may be reduced and the accompanying aching and pain may be alleviated. The application of external pressure may also lead to an improvement in venous valve function.

Prevention of the development of oedema and improvements in the action of the calf muscle pump may also be possible, even with garments that produce only limited raised pressure at the ankle.

Compression may be achieved with bandages or with graduated compression hosiery. However, when a bandage is applied to the limb it is difficult to gauge what pressure is being exerted. Bandages may also be cosmetically unacceptable to patients. Tubular bandages are not appropriate when graduated compression is required.

Venous leg ulcers

Leg ulcers are a common and recurring problem. They occur in 1.5–3 per 1000 of the general population, increasing to about 20 per 1000 in those over 80 years of age. Leg ulcers are strongly associated with venous disease, but a fifth of patients have arterial disease, either alone or in conjunction with venous disease. Patients with arterial disease must be distinguished from those with venous disease, as their management differs. The use of compression hosiery in patients with arterial disease should be avoided, as it may cause necrosis and further ulceration; in severe cases amputation may be necessary. Compression hosiery should be used with caution in those with diabetes mellitus or rheumatoid arthritis, as these patients are susceptible to small vessel disease.

Most leg ulcers are managed in the primary care setting by GPs and community nurses. Compression therapy is the treatment of choice for most venous leg ulcers. The ulcerated area should be kept clean and debrided if necessary. Although dressings are not thought to enhance healing, they are useful to absorb exudate, control odour, relieve pain and promote re-epithelialisation. Compression may be applied in the form of compression bandages, graduated compression hosiery or both. Graduated compression hosiery has been shown to aid healing of venous ulcers. It is thought that it may also help to prevent recurrence, although evidence of the latter is more limited. There is some evidence that pentoxifylline used with compression therapy may be beneficial in ulcer healing. Topical applications should be avoided if possible, but metronidazole cream or gel and activated charcoal dressings are helpful in reducing odour in heavily colonised ulcers.

Prophylaxis of postoperative deep vein thrombosis

Deep vein thrombosis (DVT) in the lower limb and pelvic veins may occur following prolonged immobility after surgery or a medical illness. Graduated compression hosiery has been shown to reduce the incidence of DVTs in these patients. Antiembolism stockings (TED stockings) may be used for this purpose, but these are not allowed on NHS prescription.

Oedema

Oedema is a characteristic of several disease states, including heart failure, renal impairment and various malignancies (often due to lymphatic obstruction). Where possible, the underlying cause of the oedema should be identified and treated. However, in many patients oedema persists, and the use of graduated compression hosiery may be beneficial.

Lymphoedema is a chronic swelling that occurs because of inadequate lymph drainage. It may be due to congenital abnormalities of the lymphatic system or to damage to this system following infection, malignancy, surgery or radiation. The management of lymphoedema has four main components:

- Skin care to reduce the risk of infection and to maintain the condition of the tissue
- External support/compression to reduce lymph formation and encourage lymph drainage
- Exercise to maximise lymph drainage
- Lymphatic drainage proximal to the swelling to stimulate drainage and to siphon away from the oedematous region.

Specialist garments are available to provide support/compression for patients with lymphoedema, but these are not available on NHS prescription.

Standards for graduated compression hosiery

A British Standard (BS 6612) for graduated compression hosiery was introduced in July 1985. Its introduction was made possible by the development of a suitable testing device, the Hosiery and Allied Trades Association (HATRA) hose pressure tester. Previously, the degree of compression exerted by individual garments could not be reliably assessed and the manufacture of hosiery was largely empirically based. The degree of pressure exerted by a garment can now be accurately defined.

The British Standard specifies that graduated compression hosiery must exert a minimum pressure of 6 mmHg at the ankle when the patient is standing, and that the degree of compression must decrease up the leg in order to prevent the garment exerting a tourniquet effect.

Hosiery compression profiles are defined in terms of the pressure exerted by garments at the ankle and the relative pressures at the calf and thigh, as outlined in Table 4.1.

Table 4.1 Pressure exerted by garments at the ankle and the relative pressures at the calf and thigh

Ankle compression value (mmHg)	Proportion of ankle compression at calf (%)	Proportion of calf compression at thigh (%)
6–10	<100	<100
11–18	80 max	85 max
19 and over	70 max	70 max

No upper limit is specified in the British Standard for ankle pressure. However, it is recognised that pressures of 40 mmHg and more may prevent arterial blood from reaching the distal part of the limb.

In addition to defining the pressure requirements, BS 6612 also states that the garment must be capable of exerting at least 85% of its original pressure after having been washed 30 times. The expected life of each garment is at least three or four months.

Types of graduated compression hosiery

Historically, a bewildering array of garments was available, some of which are listed below:

- Two-way stretch, standard elastic yarn, circular knit, nylon
- One-way stretch, seamless fine thread
- Lightweight elastic net (closed or open heel).

The introduction of British Standard 6612 considerably simplified the range of product categories. Garments are now classified according to the mean pressure exerted at the ankle, as described in Table 4.2.

Table 4.2 Classification of garments according to mean pressure exerted at the ankle

Class I	Mean ankle compression 14–17 mmHg (formerly lightweight elastic yarn). These garments are used for light or mild support in cases of early or superficial varices. They are also used for prophylaxis and treatment of varicose veins in pregnancy
Class II	Mean ankle compression 18–24 mmHg (formerly standard elastic yarn). These garments provide medium support for the treatment of mild oedema, the prevention and treatment of ulceration, and for varicosities occurring during pregnancy. They can also be used after surgery or sclerotherapy
Class III	Mean ankle compression 25–35 mmHg (formerly known as one-way stretch). Class III garments provide the strong support necessary for gross varices, severe oedema, and venous insufficiency after deep vein thrombosis. They can also be used with dressings in the treatment of chronic leg ulceration, and for the prevention and recurrence of such ulcers

The range of garments has also been simplified (Figure 4.2). Previously, anklets, kneecaps, leggings, below-knee stockings, above-knee stockings and thigh stockings were available, although not all were

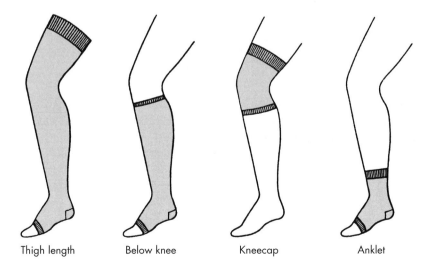

Thigh length   Below knee   Kneecap   Anklet

Figure 4.2 Graduated compression hosiery garments.

available in all materials or special types of knits. The garments available for use in the prevention and treatment of varicose veins are now restricted to thigh stockings and below-knee stockings.

Anklets (socks) and kneecaps are also available in class II and class III compression profiles, although they are supplied primarily for sports injuries, strains and other non-varicose conditions.

Garments may be fully footed or have open heels or toes. The use of modern fibres has also increased the range of hosiery colours. Darker shades are now available, and these may encourage compliance in men as the garments are virtually indistinguishable from socks.

Hosiery accessories

Most garments are manufactured with a more highly elasticated portion at the upper end as an aid to keeping the hosiery in position. As tights cannot be prescribed by doctors, the use of a suspender belt (Figure 4.3) may be needed to ensure that thigh-length stockings stay in place during normal exercise. Some women may already possess a suspender belt which can be used for this purpose. For those who do not, and for men prescribed thigh-length garments, a one-size suspender belt is available. The belt consists of a rigid, two-piece waistband with adjustable fastening. Four suspenders are sewn to the outside of the waistband.

An alternative usually more acceptable to men is the Y-shaped suspender, which can be fastened to buttons sewn in the trouser lining. The forked ends hang downwards to the top of the stocking. Suspenders are

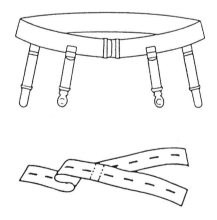

Figure 4.3 Suspenders for graduated compression hosiery.

automatically supplied for any thigh-length garment for men, but the doctor must order them separately for women.

Selecting the correct hosiery

The choice of the appropriate graduated compression garment depends on the indication, the area affected, and whether the patient is male or female. The doctor may order the garment in terms of the degree of compression required (mild, moderate or strong) or by the compression class (I, II, or III/1, 2 or 3).

Severe varicosities require a greater degree of compression than mild varicosities. The choice of the correct garment is determined by the position of the varicosities. The garment should preferably reach the highest level of the varices and extend at least 5 cm above that level.

Whereas the choice previously lay between nylon-covered or cotton-covered garments, the introduction of modern materials has limited the choice primarily to colours. Even when hosiery is concealed (e.g. beneath trousers) dark shades may be more appropriate for men, so that even thigh-length garments give the outward appearance of ordinary socks.

Measuring and selecting the correct size of hosiery

In all cases, the usefulness of the hosiery product is entirely dependent on the accuracy of the limb measurements and the correct selection of garments based on those measurements. The following guidelines will ensure that the correct garment is chosen:

- Measurements should be taken as early in the morning as possible, preferably before the patient has been standing for long or taken any exercise. These precautions ensure that the leg has not swollen. If such precautions are not practicable and the patient has walked to the pharmacy, the limb should be rested in a horizontal position for as long as possible before the measurements are taken.
- All manufacturers produce diagrams to indicate the number and position of measurements necessary for satisfactory fitting. Circumference measurements are commonly taken at the top of the thigh (for thigh-length stockings only), the knee, the calf and the ankle. The length of the foot may also be included.
- Measurements should be taken next to the skin and should be accurate to the nearest 5 mm; they should not be taken from old garments. Measurements should be taken starting at the top of the

limb and working downwards, to prevent undue concern to the patient about where the highest measurement may be. A female member of staff should be present if a male pharmacist is measuring a female patient.

Measurements must not be adjusted to take into account differences in the pressure required to be exerted along the garment. All pressure differences are incorporated into the hosiery during manufacture. If a pair of garments is ordered, individual measurements of each limb must be taken. Most healthy legs can vary slightly in diameter and such differences may be accentuated by the presence of varicosities of varying severity. Each time a new prescription is issued the patient should be measured, as changes in size may occur.

When the measurements have been recorded, manufacturers' charts should be consulted. Most charts give a range of values (in centimetres or inches, or both) for the individual measurement points. The correct size of garment can be selected by choosing the size within whose ranges all the measurements lie (Figure 4.4). For example, a patient's measurements for the points on the Scholl Ultima chart shown here might be: A – 45 cm; B – 34 cm; C – 25 cm; D – 24.5 cm. Although measurements A and B could apply to small and medium sizes, measurements C and D clearly fall exclusively within the ranges of the medium-sized garment, and this would be the appropriate size.

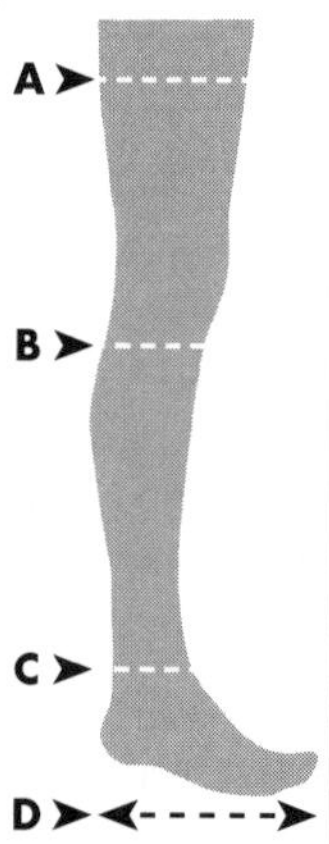

SIZE	S	M	L	XL
A	16"–20" 40.5cm–52cm	17"–21" 43cm–54cm	19"–23" 48cm–59.5cm	21"–25" 53cm–65cm
B	12"–14" 30.5cm–36.5cm	13"–15" 33cm–39cm	14"–16" 35.5cm–41.5cm	15"–17" 38cm–44cm
C	7¾"–9¼" 19.5cm–24.5cm	8½"–10" 21.5cm–26.5cm	9¼"–10¾" 23.5cm–28.5cm	10"–11¾" 25.5cm–30.5cm
D	8"–8½" 20.5cm–22.5cm	9"–9½" 23cm–25cm	10"–10½" 25.5cm–27.5cm	10½"–11¾" 26.5cm–30.5cm

Figure 4.4 Scholl Ultima measuring chart for graduated compression hosiery (courtesy of Scholl).

In 95% of cases the measurements taken are likely to conform to one of the stock sizes produced by a manufacturer. Where the measurements are significantly different, garments must be made to measure. Made-to-measure garments are available in all three compression classes.

Despite improvements in the appearance and comfort of graduated compression hosiery compliance is still poor. It may be helpful to reinforce the importance of wearing the garment and to discuss any concerns the patient may have.

Fitting and removing hosiery

If the garment is fitted with confidence and ease, any apprehension the patient may have over wearing the hosiery could be reduced. Correct fitting is also essential to ensure the maximum life of the garment. The sequence of events in fitting and removing the garment is illustrated in Figure 4.5, and the following points should be taken into consideration:

• Everyday hose should be removed and, if required, the leg may be lightly coated with powder.
• The patient should remove all sharp objects (e.g. rings and bracelets) and trim long and rough nails on both fingers and toes.
• The garment should be turned inside-out as far as the heel pouch. The heel should be laid flat so that the foot may slip in easily and the toes and heel be correctly positioned.
• The rest of the garment should be eased over the foot and ankle, ensuring that it does not become bunched at any one point as severe discomfort may result. The garment may then be gently pulled up the leg, but care should be taken not to damage the fibres with the fingers or nails.

Stocking aids are available for patients who find it difficult to put their stockings on, but these are not allowed on NHS prescription.

Removing the hosiery is usually easier than putting it on. The garment should be peeled down as far as the ankle, in effect turning it inside-out. It can then be removed from the leg by gently pulling the toe portion.

Care of graduated compression hosiery

If the manufacturer's instructions for fitting and removing graduated compression hosiery are followed, garments may have a useful life of up

- Turn hosiery inside out, leaving foot section tucked in
- Place patient's foot on your knees
- If fitting an open-toe stocking, place a fitting socklet over the foot to help the stocking slide on to the foot.

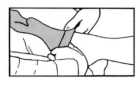 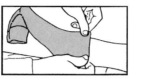 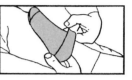

- Place the first two fingers of each hand inside the foot of the stocking, ease the stocking on to the patient's foot and slide it over the ankle as far as it will go without using undue force
- Stretch the stocking up the leg from the ankle in short sections of 1–2 inches at a time using a slight twisting action

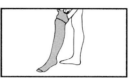

- When the stocking is fitted up to the knee invite the patient to stand and ask them to continue pulling the stocking from the knee to the thigh in the same way
- The patient should then fasten the stocking to the suspenders

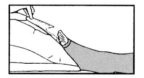

- If used, the fitting socklet should now be removed

Figure 4.5 Fitting the garment (adapted from Scholl Ultima Quick Step Measuring and Fitting Guide, with kind permission of Scholl).

to three months. Prolonged use may lead to a gradual reduction in the compression exerted and the support provided.

Washing instructions must also be followed carefully. Garments should generally be hand-washed in lukewarm water (40°C) with pure soap-flakes, not detergent. Some garments may be suitable for gentle machine washing (according to manufacturer's recommendations). Temperatures in excess of 50°C may denature the elastane fibres. Excess water in the garment can be removed by folding the stocking and gently squeezing it. Under no circumstances should it be wrung out or twisted, as this can damage the material. Garments should be dried flat, away from direct heat sources. They should not be hung vertically from a washing line and, when dry, should not be ironed.

If the original packaging in which the garment was supplied has been lost, washing instructions may be found on the upper portion of the hosiery.

Prescribing information

The prescriber must specify the following information on a prescription for graduated compression hosiery:

- The quantity of garments required: single (right or left)/pair
- Type of garment: e.g. thigh-length stocking
- Compression class: I, II, or III
- Accessories (if required).

Further reading

Foord-Kelcy G (2001). *Guidelines – Summarising Clinical Guidelines for Primary Care*, Vol 13. Berkhamsted: Medendium Group Publishing.

Haynes B, Glasziou P (2001). *Evidence-based Medicine*. London: BMJ Publishing.

National Pharmaceutical Association (1999). *NPA Guide to the Drug Tariff and NHS Dispensing for England and Wales*. St Albans: National Pharmaceutical Association.

NHS Centre for Reviews and Dissemination, University of York. *Effective health care: compression therapy for venous leg ulcers*. 1997; 3: 1–12.

5

Wound healing and wound management products

Sarah ME Cockbill

A wound can be defined as any process that leads to the disruption of the normal architecture of a tissue. A fundamental theorem in the study of wound healing is that 'all wounds are not the same'. They may be closed (contusions, bruises, ruptures, sprains) or open (abrasions, lacerations, avulsions, ballistic, penetrating, hernias, and excised or surgical wounds). Open wounds are by far the most common and are characterised by a break in the skin. The process of wound healing depends on the type of tissue damaged and the nature of the tissue disruption. Deep open wounds in bone do not heal in the same way or at the same rate as super-ficial epithelial wounds, largely because bone 'tissue' consists of up to 65% inorganic calcium-based matrix.

The objective of any wound management regimen is to heal the wound in the shortest time possible and with minimal pain, discomfort and scarring to the patient. Success in fulfilling the objective will be assisted by an understanding of the healing process and a knowledge of the contributions that the existing range of wound management products can make to initiating and maintaining the optimal micro-environment for healing.

The process of healing is the replacement of damaged tissue by new living material, with the intended reconstruction of the original structure. However, unlike certain other less highly evolved and specialised forms of life, humans can regenerate very few tissues, with the partial exception of epidermal cells. Wound healing is accompanied by the formation of a permanent new structure lacking functional ability, the scar.

Structure of the skin

The skin is the largest organ of the body and consists of a complex three-tiered structure (Figure 5.1). Its function is protective. It covers the other organs, plays a role in temperature regulation, allows the removal of waste products, incorporates sensors for the detection of pain, external pressures and external temperature changes, absorbs sunlight (thus aiding its conversion to vitamin D), and acts as a waterproof barrier. The skin is composed of several layers: the outer epidermis and stratum corneum, which protect against injury and contamination; the dermis, which contains the capillary network that provides nutrients and removes waste; the sensors for detecting pain and immediate environmental changes; and the subcutis, from which the dermis and epidermis develop. The stratum corneum also acts as a barrier to the loss of water from the body. Its destruction is an important contributory factor to the development of shock in severely burnt patients. Skin also contains sebaceous glands, hair follicles and sweat glands.

The cornified cells on the surface of the skin do not contain blood vessels or nerve endings but consist of keratin, which is continuously shed as squames. About 1 g of keratinised cells is shed each day as dandruff. Shed cells are replaced by new cells produced by the basal layer, and these continuously migrate to the surface of the skin. The thickness of the epidermal layer varies from a thin membrane at internal flexures (e.g. at the elbow) to thick, compacted layers at points that bear considerable pressure (e.g. the palms and soles). The epidermal layer is crossed by hair follicles, sebaceous glands and sweat glands which arise in the dermis.

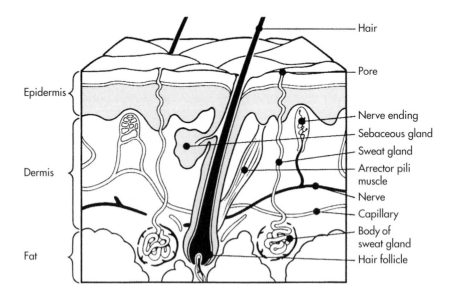

Figure 5.1 Structure of the skin.

The outer surface of the dermis (the papillary layer) is formed of ridges that project into the epidermis. The papillary layer contains blood vessels, lymphatics and nerve endings. The blood supply is distributed between outer vessels, which nourish the epidermal cells, and deeper vessels, which lie just outside the lower subcutaneous layer of fat. The elasticity of skin, and its ability to retain and lose water rapidly, is the consequence of the presence of a network of collagen fibres. The dermis also contains sweat glands unevenly distributed over the body. Thick skin contains a high proportion of eccrine glands, which secrete sweat throughout life. The apocrine glands, which remain inactive until puberty, are located in the axillary, breast and pubic regions. The bacterial decomposition of their exudate produces the unpleasant characteristic odour of the adult.

Beneath the dermis is the fat-containing subcutaneous layer, which is highly vascularised. It insulates internal structures from excessive heat and reduces heat loss in cold climates. Its spongy texture and flexibility may also dissipate the effects of physical trauma.

Classification of wounds

Wounds may be classified according to the number of skin layers affected and whether tissue has been lost. Simple surgical incisions do not involve loss of tissue. Conversely, traumatic wounds (e.g. lacerations and abrasions) and chronic wounds (e.g. burns and varicose ulcers) are frequently accompanied by varying degrees of tissue loss. A superficial wound that will heal rapidly by regeneration of epithelial cells comprises damage limited to the epithelial tissue (epidermis). A partial-thickness wound involves the deeper dermal layer and includes vessel damage. Its repair process is more complex. A full-thickness wound affects the subcutaneous fat layer and beyond. Its healing requires the synthesis of new connective tissue and takes longer because it contracts, whereas partial-thickness wounds do not.

In the management of wounds and the use of wound management products, further classification of wounds as clean and non-infected is essential. Contaminated wounds should never be closed without thorough removal of all the damaged tissue (debridement). It may also be necessary to delay closure until the risk of infection has receded.

The process of wound healing

Healing by primary intention

If the two apposed surfaces of a clean, incised wound (which has not been subject to a significant degree of tissue loss) are held together, healing will take place from the internal layers outwards. The two surfaces may be held together by sutures, wound management products or surface adhesives. The process of healing by primary intention is initiated by the movement of epithelial cells from the two edges of the wound towards its centre. They usually meet and commence interlocking within four to seven days of the incision. The reappearance of normal skin follows the keratinisation and thinning of the epidermis. The pre-trauma strength of the tissue will never be completely regained.

Healing by secondary intention

If there has been a significant loss of tissue in the formation of the wound, healing will begin with the production of granulation tissue at the base of the wound. The process of healing by secondary intention always involves contraction of the wound. The degree of contraction is greatest during the first few days after the wound has been inflicted.

The mechanism of healing may be most usefully considered chronologically, although it must be remembered that the process is continuous, and that well-defined stages do not occur in practice. The process of wound healing follows a specific sequence of phases, which may overlap.

Stages in the healing process

Wound healing is a complicated and precise series of events (Figures 5.2 and 5.3) that involves cellular, physiological, biochemical and molecular processes which result ultimately in connective tissue repair and the formation of a fibrous scar. It starts immediately after damage has occurred, but the mechanism and speed of healing and the eventual nature of the regenerated tissue depend on the type of wound. The first phase is the inflammatory (reaction) phase, which occurs as a normal part of healing immediately after the trauma. This is followed by the proliferative (repair) phase and finally by the maturation (regeneration) phase.

Stage 1: the inflammatory (reaction) phase

Inflammation is a protective tissue response to an injury that is the beginning of the healing process. It is characterised by pain, heat, redness,

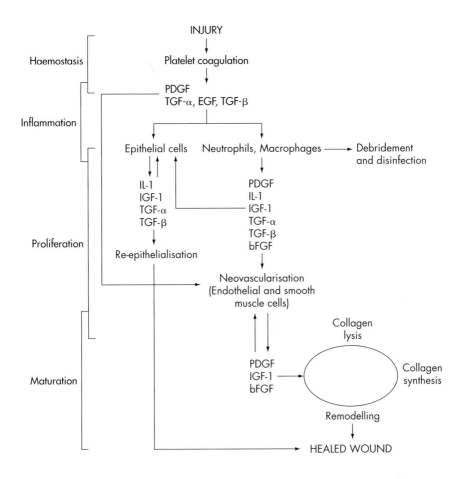

Figure 5.2 Proposed interaction of endogenous growth factors following injury to epithelium and underlying connective tissue.

swelling and loss of function at the site of the wound. These classic signs of inflammation can be seen almost immediately after an injury, and are also characteristic of an impending wound infection. They are outward signs of damage and result from vasodilatation caused by the secretion of histamine and enzymes from damaged tissue, and from the passage of plasma into the affected area owing to increased capillary permeability (diapedesis). The plasma transports antibodies, leucocytes (particularly polymorphs), growth factors, macrophages and fibroblasts to the site of damage. These elements start the repair process by clearing debris and damaged tissue by phagocytosis. The purpose is to destroy, dilute or isolate the injurious agent and the injured tissues.

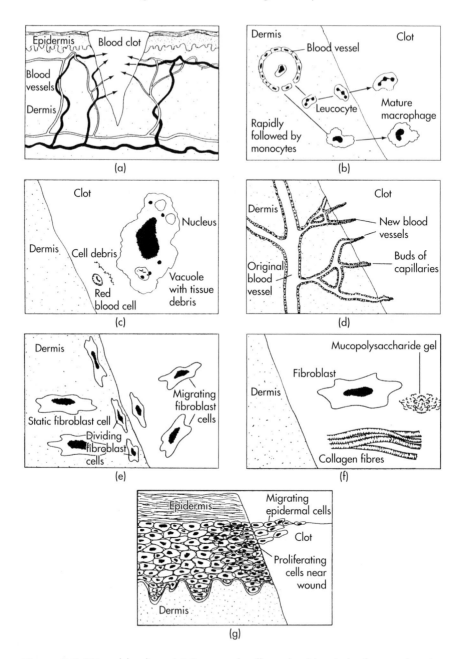

Figure 5.3 Wound healing. (a) Damaged cells and a blood clot form within the wound. (b) The blood clot is invaded by leucocytes. (c) The debris is cleared by macrophages. (d) Regeneration starts with the growth of new blood cells. (e) The clot is invaded by fibroblasts from connective tissue. (f) Gels and fibres are formed as a result of fibroblast activity. (g) Regrowth of the epidermis starts.

The drop in potential difference across the edges of the wound after injury acts as the stimulant for Hagemann factor XII, which is responsible for activating the healing cascade. The effector systems within the cascade – the plasminogen cascade, the complement cascade, the kinin cascade and the clotting cascade – interlink to control infection and regenerate tissue. They release chemical mediators (e.g. complement C5a), fibrin degradation factors, platelet activity factors and vasoconstrictors (e.g. histamine and serotonin).

Initially, cessation of blood flow from the wound is achieved by vasoconstriction at the wound site and clot formation. Immediately following injury, platelets aggregate and release coagulation factors and growth factors that are vital for haemostasis and initiation of the healing process. The platelets that form the clot are activated by exposure to collagen or microfibrils and to platelet-derived growth factor (PDGF) produced by the erythrocytes damaged during injury. Platelets adhere to the subendothelium exposed after injury, flatten and release a prostaglandin which encourages aggregation and, in combination with vasoconstrictors (histamine and serotonin from mast cells), reduce immediate blood loss prior to the initiation of the clotting cascade. Activated platelets release several growth factors: PDGF, platelet-derived epidermal growth factor (PDEGF), epidermal growth factor (EGF), transforming growth factors α and β (TGF-α, TGF-β), heparin-binding epidermal growth factor (HB-EGF) and insulin-like growth factor-1 (IGF-1). These stimulate cell growth and migration at the injured site from within their α granules. These growth factors stimulate the sequential migration of cells (neutrophils, then macrophages, then fibroblasts) into the wound site. Activated platelets also stimulate the intrinsic coagulation system, which converts fibrinogen to a fibrin mesh to produce a thrombus that stabilises the platelet plug.

The clot maintains haemostasis and creates a provisional matrix for the migration of cells (monocytes, fibroblasts and keratinocytes) to the wound, with the consequent release of their cytokines and mediators. When blood flow is controlled, vasoconstriction is replaced by vasodilatation. This allows the influx of a protein-rich exudate containing antibodies, various complement fractions, and other substances essential to the healing process (e.g. growth factors and cytokines).

Vasodilation is accompanied by increased vascular permeability, which results in plasma entering the site of injury via diapedesis. Oedema is observed, together with an increase in wound temperature and pain caused by the action of histamine, kinins and prostaglandins. This permeability may last up to one hour. The occlusion of the local wound lymphatic channels by fibrin prevents the spread of the inflammation. During inflammation, white blood cells (neutrophils) migrate to the wound area and, with macrophages, ingest bacteria and cell debris by phagocytosis. The successful macrophage function normally indicates the end of the acute inflammatory reaction.

The chemoattractants released by the platelets stimulate the rapid influx of neutrophils and monocytes from the circulation to the wound site by diapedesis. Neutrophils and monocytes have a common origin (a pluripotent bone marrow stem cell) and overlapping functions. Once the monocyte becomes phagocytic, it is referred to as a macrophage. Both macrophages and neutrophils can kill and digest bacteria and damaged tissue and thus help prevent infection by microorganisms that may be introduced into the host through the wound. Neutrophils are short-lived and die once they have phagocytosed bacteria and necrotic tissue. However, they continue to aid healing as they release toxins which further stimulate the inflammatory response and contribute to the activation that produces macrophages from monocytes. Macrophages also serve as an important source of growth factors that regulate the wound healing response.

Growth factors and cytokines are polypeptides transiently produced by cells. They exert their hormone-like function on other cells via specific cell-surface receptors. Their activities overlap, and the effect of most of them depends on the group and pattern of regulatory molecules to which the cell is exposed. Growth factors are so named because of their stimulatory effect on cell proliferation. They display both stimulatory and inhibitory activities, even within the same cell, depending on the state of activation and differentiation of the cells and the presence of other stimulating factors.

Macrophages are pivotal in bringing about the first stages of healing. Subsequently, they control and direct it before finally stopping it when the repair is complete. These cells modulate the immune response by induction of lipoxygenase products through stimulation of the arachidonic acid cascade. In addition to aiding debridement at the wound site, they are involved in the secretion and synthesis of the collagenases (neutrophil elastase and matrix metalloproteinase eight (MMP 8)) preparatory to laying down a new extracellular matrix (connective tissue). They are another source of the growth factors PDGF and TGF-β, and regulate fibroblast migration and proliferation by production of the cytokine interleukin-1β (IL-1β).

Stage 2: the repair phase

Proliferation

The inflammation phase, which overlaps the proliferation or repair phase, begins with a period of cellular proliferation. During the transition from inflammation to proliferation, the number of inflammatory cells decreases and the number of fibroblasts within the wound site increases. Fibroblasts are attached to the site and synthesise collagen, beginning on the fourth or fifth day of injury and continuing for two to four weeks. Capillaries are formed by endothelial budding, with the production of granulation tissue and lysis of the previously produced fibrin network. Specific chemoattractants (growth factors TGF-β and PDGF) stimulate the influx of macrophages. At the surface of the wound, epithelial cells begin to cover the tissue defect. The end of this phase is marked by the re-epithelialisation of the wound surface.

The first stage of this process is to restore vascular integrity (angiogenesis) and involves the migration, proliferation and organisation of endothelial cells under the influence of the following growth factors: acidic fibroblast growth factor (aFGF), tumour necrosis factor-β (TNF-β), wound angiogenesis factor (WAF), vascular endothelial growth factor (VEGF) and EGF. The regeneration of capillaries and arterioles continues until equilibrium of arterial and venous blood pressure is obtained within the microcirculation. Endothelial cells are organised so that developing tissues are assured a supply of oxygen and nutrients. This is achieved as capillary loops infiltrate into the wound space.

Also during this phase, extracellular matrix (ECM) components are deposited to replace lost or damaged tissue. Connective tissue is synthesised and is known initially as granulation tissue. This happens around day four of healing.

Granulation tissue is composed of macrophages, fibroblasts and neovasculature in a loose matrix which is subsequently covered by an epithelium. The macrophages produce cytokines, which stimulate cells to activate fibroblasts to protein synthesis and to proliferation, activate endothelial cells to make adhesion factors and various mediators, and to activate T and B cells.

Fibroblasts are the major cells responsible for the production of tropocollagen, the precursor to collagen, elastin, and the proteoglycans that make up the ECM in connective tissue. Fibroblasts also secrete a range of growth factors which play a part in this phase of the wound healing process: insulin-like growth factor one (IGF-1), basic fibroblast growth factor (bFGF), TGF-β, and keratinocyte growth factor (KGF).

bFGF and PDGF stimulate connective tissue formation and directly enhance epithelialisation. EGF and TGF-β increase the rate of epithelialisation, and KGF stimulates keratinocyte proliferation. Epithelial cells adjacent to the wound site are also an important source of these growth factors. Fibroblasts, as well as macrophages, are a major source of matrix metalloproteinases (MMPs), which degrade the ECM at an appropriate time, and also of tissue inhibitors of MMPs (TIMPs), which are proteolytic enzymes responsible for the elimination of fibres that do not contribute to the structural strength of the wound.

As granulation is completed the wound edges contract, thereby reducing the size of the defect. This is achieved by the transformation of fibroblasts to myofibroblasts, which contain contractile proteins. The degree of contraction varies with the depth of the wound. Vascularity is reduced and the inflammatory cells leave the healing site. Usually a fine-line scar results.

The activity of the macrophages and polymorphs continues in all damaged tissues irrespective of their degree of vascularisation up to the fifth post-trauma day. Even if the wound is clean and the number of polymorphs is consequently reduced, repair mechanisms will continue. However, if the number of macrophages is reduced, healing will cease. This is thought to be a consequence of the directing role that macrophages undertake and of their involvement in the production of fibroblasts which synthesise the body's principal structural protein, collagen. The presence of collagen may be detected in fresh wounds from as early as the second day.

Macrophages also stimulate new blood vessels from the surrounding tissue to grow into the wound. Their appearance heralds the next stage of healing.

Organisation

Depending on the severity of the wound and its site, the proliferative phase may begin as early as the third day and last until the end of the third week. This phase marks the period of regain of order within the wound, with the production of collagen reaching a peak from about day five to day seven. Fibroblasts act as the source of new collagen, with the greatest production occurring in a slightly acidic environment. The importance of adequate nutrition in a patient at this stage is critical, as the presence of vitamin C acts as an important stimulator of collagen manufacture. In its absence, newly formed blood vessels remain unsupported and subsequently break down, producing the characteristic appearance of purpura.

Endothelial cells produce buds, which fuse and subsequently differentiate into blood vessels (i.e. arterioles, capillaries and venules). In an adequately nourished patient these vessels are supported within the scaffolding of collagen fibres, producing granulation tissue. The amount of granulation correlates directly with the extent of inflammation that occurred in stage 1 of the healing process. This in turn depends on how effectively dead tissue, foreign bodies and infection have been excluded from the wound site. The importance of a clean environment, a healthy immune response and a well-nourished individual cannot be overstressed. The overproduction of granulation tissue will result in an outsized and usually unsightly scar.

Stage 3: the maturation/regeneration phase

This is the longest stage of wound healing and can last from three weeks to two years after the original injury. This phase overlaps with the repair phase and consists of a series of dynamic processes in which the ECM composition continually reflects a balance between synthesis and degradation of the components present in the wound. Fibroblasts produce tropocollagen molecules which combine to form collagen fibrils, filaments and fibres. There is an increase in the tensile strength of the wound which, in cavity wounds, is accompanied by contraction caused by myofibroblasts. As collagen is deposited the fibroblasts disappear. The wound will now be covered by epidermis and the maturation will continue for up to two years, with the period varying between individuals and their age at the time of injury. Fibroblasts continue to be important, as they are responsible for the deposition of matrix materials and are the source of MMPs and TIMPs (see above).

Collagen type III synthesised during granulation is replaced by collagen type I, which is stronger and gives the tissue greater tensile strength. As this collagen develops, there is a decreased demand for oxygen and nutrients within the wound and therefore a reduction in the microvasculature. The new tissue that develops is known as scar tissue, and this will only ever reach between 70 and 80% of the original tissue strength.

In addition to the mechanisms described above, two other processes must be considered, particularly if there has been a loss of tissue in the formation of a wound.

Contraction

Wound contraction is a natural healing process which allows open wounds to heal almost as rapidly as those that have been sutured.

Contraction appears to be mediated by myofibroblasts which contain smooth muscle fibrils, although the process is not universally effective. Wounds on the abdomen and on the back of the neck contract considerably, leaving only small scars. Those that are inflicted on the lower leg and on the face contract poorly, possibly owing to the close interactions of the overlying skin with many underlying structures.

Epithelialisation

Epithelialisation varies between wound types. Wounds that contain few or no epithelial cells will be subject to a longer and more difficult healing process than superficial wounds, which already contain islands of cells that proliferate rapidly. Sutured full-thickness wounds will have new epithelium within three days, although they will have little tensile strength. In partial-thickness wounds the epithelial cells from hair follicles and sebaceous glands migrate towards one another. In full-thickness wounds, in which there is a lack of dermal appendages, epithelial cells must migrate from the edges of the wound. When they meet, contact inhibition halts their lateral proliferation but they continue to proliferate vertically, to produce a multicellular layer which resurfaces the wound. The protective barrier formed is due to the migration, proliferation and differentiation of keratinocytes, which arise from the epithelium peripheral to the wound or from hair follicles. Keratinocytes, epidermal cells which secrete keratin, migrate into the area within hours of the injury. They secrete membrane components, fibronectin, collagen and laminin.

The epithelialisation process is sensitive to environmental factors such as pH, moisture and temperature. Deviation from the optimum values can have a detrimental effect. Once repair has taken place, the wound will still undergo a continued phase of regeneration or maturation. In the intervening period, however, the epidermis is unable to perform its essential role as an effective barrier to the passage of water.

Other components of the wound and its management

Necrotic tissue and debridement

The presence of yellowish-brown or blackened tissue in the wound indicates necrosis (i.e. an area of dead material). It is commonly present in pressure ulcers and it delays healing and promotes infection. Effective wound management requires its removal by the process of debridement.

Mechanical or surgical debridement involves physical removal of the dead tissue, usually by cutting with scissors or a scalpel and lifting it with forceps. The tissue may also be removed chemically, using keratolytic agents (e.g. benzoyl peroxide). Dead tissue can be selectively broken down by the use of enzymatic agents (e.g. collagenase or streptokinase), but these appear to be of lower potency than chemical agents.

Slough

The accumulation of dead cells in the exudate from wounds is a natural part of the healing process. The exudate, which appears yellowish because of the presence of leucocytes, may accumulate into an unsightly mass on the surface of the wound and is termed 'slough'. The process of its removal, providing a clean area for the regrowth of new tissue, is called desloughing. Mechanical removal may be done with a swab, an absorptive wound management product, or irrigation. Great care must be taken in the process of desloughing to prevent further inflammation and damage to the traumatised skin. In particular. the appearance of granulation tissue under the exudate must not be mistaken for unwanted slough.

Factors that influence the effectiveness of wound healing

To produce effective wound healing, the body must supply a range of materials and nutrients to the site of damage. Factors that promote healing include an adequate blood supply and a healthy diet that provides protein, vitamin A, vitamin C, zinc and copper. By inference, a nutritional, physical or clinical situation in which any one of these factors is lacking may have a deleterious effect on wound healing. Both systemic and local factors may challenge the successful continuation of the healing stages. In addition to nutritional status, the systemic factors include concurrent therapy (e.g. corticosteroids), prostaglandin inhibition, oncolytic agents and clinical conditions (e.g. anaemia and diabetes). These must be monitored and the objective must be the holistic management of the patient and not just the wound. Optimum healing can also be encouraged by the elimination from the wound of debris, which may otherwise act as an ideal environment for the multiplication of microorganisms. The presence of infection must be avoided at all costs.

Blood supply

The growing edge of new epithelium has an insatiable appetite for blood. Any reduction in the provision of an adequate blood supply slows the rate of healing considerably by reducing the levels of oxygen, cells and nutrients reaching the wound. This explains why the prevention of clinical shock is essential, both after trauma and after blood loss during surgery. Equally, a patient suffering from any disease in which the circulation is impaired (e.g. arteriosclerosis, diabetes mellitus, Raynaud's syndrome) may be less capable of rapid and effective wound healing.

Nutritional factors

A wound in a patient with a good nutritional status is likely to heal more easily and quickly than a similar wound in an undernourished individual. Poor nutrition is one reason for the notoriously slow healing of decubitus ulcers in the elderly. It may also adversely affect patients suffering from malabsorption syndromes (e.g. coeliac disease), colitis and malignant disease. The important role of vitamins in wound healing has also been mentioned briefly. Vitamin C is required for collagen synthesis, and it has been shown that plasma levels of the vitamin decrease after injury. Vitamin A is required for the cross-linking of collagen and the proliferation of epithelial cells. Vitamin A levels in the blood and liver are reduced after certain types of injury (e.g. burns).

Roles for zinc and copper in wound healing have been postulated. Zinc is required for protein synthesis and is a cofactor in enzymatic reactions. Demand for zinc increases during cell proliferation and protein secretion, and therefore deficiencies of zinc may retard epithelialisation and collagen synthesis. It is also thought that zinc affects the immune system and has an inhibitory action on bacterial growth. Supplements given to well-nourished individuals do not appear to speed the rate of healing, and research is ongoing to establish the level of serum zinc depletion below which zinc supplementation would be beneficial. Copper, on the other hand, is required for the cross-linking of collagen fibres.

Drugs

The importance of inflammation in the mechanism of wound healing was originally thought to contraindicate the use of anti-inflammatory drugs after trauma. However, it has been shown that therapeutic doses of most of these drugs do not retard wound healing, but may in fact reduce both pain and pyrexia.

The use of corticosteroids has been equally controversial. In large doses they have been shown to suppress wound healing and reduce the effectiveness of the body's ability to respond to infection. Conversely, the stress the body undergoes during injury results in the production of large quantities of endogenous steroids, and this is thought to have little or no effect on the efficiency of healing.

The use of cytotoxic drugs poses significant problems in the treatment of patients who have undergone surgery to remove malignancies. Not only do these agents interfere with the process of cell replication (e.g. in the re-epithelialisation of a wound), they also attentuate the defence mechanisms of the body, rendering it liable to infection. Equally, the strength of any new tissue formed is considerably reduced in the presence of cytotoxic drugs.

Infection

The presence of infective bacteria in wounds is extremely common and prolongs the time required for wound healing. Decreased fibroblast activity in the presence of bacteria and the encouragement of leucocytes to release lysozymes, which destroy newly formed collagen, can delay healing. Additionally, the presence of multiplying microorganisms may ensure that there is competition for the available nutrients.

Infections are commonly limited to subcutaneous tissue, particularly fat. However, some may also produce systemic effects, causing a reduction in the general state of health of the patient and possibly harmful psychological effects from the sight and smell of a purulent malodorous wound. The most common causative organisms are *Clostridium* spp., *Streptococcus* spp., *Staphylococcus* spp., *Escherichia coli*, and *Pseudomonas* spp.

The main prerequisite for the successful resolution of wound infection is adequate drainage, which in some cases will require an additional incision. The use of systemic antibiotics may assist in eliminating the infection, but the use of topical antimicrobials remains controversial.

Hypergranulation

During healing the wound becomes progressively filled with granulation tissue until the base of the original cavity is almost level with the surrounding skin. At this stage the epithelium around the wound margin begins to grow over the surface of the wound, restoring the integrity of the epidermis. Occasionally the production of granulation tissue continues after the wound cavity has been filled, leading to the formation of hypergranulation tissue or 'proud flesh'. This is sometimes associated with the use of occlusive wound management materials. It can be removed either with a caustic agent (e.g. a silver nitrate pencil) or by the short-term application of a corticosteroid cream or ointment under medical supervision.

Oedema

An excess quantity of intracellular fluid reduces the effectiveness of tissue metabolism and delays wound healing. Oedema may be a consequence of any condition in which venous return is impaired (e.g. heart failure, leg ulcers, pressure ulcers). Appropriate measures include the administration of diuretics, the use of elastic hosiery, and encouraging the patient to exercise and to continue to be mobile.

Incontinence

Faecal or urinary incontinence may act as a factor in the development of pressure and decubitus ulceration. The skin rapidly becomes macerated, and the urine and faeces also act as a source of bacterial infection. Close attention to cleaning and drying the skin is essential to allow efficient wound healing.

Properties of an ideal wound management product

Optimal conditions must be created within and around a wound to obtain effective and efficient wound healing. These vary according to the site, type and depth of the wound, and associated physiological and pathological factors. However, an ideal wound management product may be proposed to meet the requirements of the majority of wounds.

Local factors which delay healing may be avoided by providing products that produce the optimal microenvironment for healing. Passive products such as gauzes and absorbents (e.g. absorbent cotton and Gamgee tissue) plug and conceal wounds and were originally extensively used, but contributed nothing to the healing process. However, in 1959, Melolin (Smith & Nephew Healthcare Ltd) was developed and marketed as the first 'non-adherent' dressing. Since that time there have been both technological and clinical advances in the design and use of dressing materials. These developments have resulted in more successful management of soft tissue injuries of different aetiologies, and have led to the present range of interactive and bioactive dressings. Interactive dressings maintain the optimum microenvironment for wound healing at the surface of the wound; bioactive dressings potentiate the healing cascade in different wounds. This microenvironment should be moist at the wound interface, but remove excess exudate to avoid irritation and excoriation.

The tissue temperature should be maintained and the injury protected from infective microorganisms, foreign particles and toxic compounds. In addition, when the dressing is changed there should be no secondary trauma due to adherence.

Interactive dressings are individually designed to meet the different environmental stages found in the three wound healing phases. No single dressing will meet all the criteria required in all of the healing stages. Careful selection based on knowledge and experience is necessary if rapid healing is to be achieved with minimal discomfort to the patient. In the future, bioactive products (e.g. growth factors) which have a cellular activity and are used to potentiate one or more steps in the healing cascade will be further developed for use in wound management.

Traditional wound management products

Traditional passive wound management materials were developed and used on an empirical basis, and the range of products available changed little until recently. Historically, a 'dressing' has been described as a material which covers a wound to allow healing to take place. Little thought was given to the interaction between the dressing and the processes of wound healing. The dressing was used as a passive agent, mainly intended to protect the wound, keep it warm and hide its unpleasant appearance. Equally, a 'bandage' was an agent commonly used to keep a dressing in place at the site of the trauma, to immobilise a damaged area, or to compress the wound and the surrounding area. Many of these traditional products are still in use today, but significant advances have been made through the development of modern interactive wound management products.

Although considerable individual variations may exist, passive wound management materials can be regarded as consisting of three main components:

- A wound-facing layer. Absorbent wound-facing layers remove excess exudate, although the attraction of the dressing material for the exudate frequently causes the material to adhere to the wound. Examples include absorbent gauze, muslin and lint. Non-absorbent materials may be produced by impregnating the absorbent material (e.g. gauze) with a fat-based agent (e.g. yellow soft paraffin).

- Absorbent layer. If the wound is producing large quantities of exudate it may pass through the wound-facing layer of the dressing into a thicker layer of greater absorbency. The absorbent layer is commonly composed of a non-woven (e.g. cotton wool or cellulose wadding) or woven material (e.g. absorbent gauzes, rayon or cotton).

- Outer layer. The outer layer is intended to provide support to the dressing, as an extensible material or a self-adhesive plaster.

Absorbents

Absorbent dressings remove excess quantities of exudate from the wound. They can be used in the form of swabs (e.g. to cleanse the skin and for the application of drugs), as an absorbent pad placed directly on the wound, or on top of a non-adherent material. The absorbent agent can be used individually (e.g. absorbent cotton) or in combination (e.g. gauze and cotton tissue). The material can be applied dry and may possess considerable absorptive capacity, or it can be moistened before use.

Materials which are produced to *British Pharmacopoeia* (BP) and *European Pharmacopoeia* (PhEur) specifications are of a higher quality than those designated as 'hospital quality'.

Adhesive dressings

Adhesive dressings, or dressing strips, may be permeable, semipermeable or occlusive. They are the main type of dressing material that the general public may keep at home for use in minor accidents. Permeable adhesive dressings include elastic adhesive dressing and permeable plastic wound dressing. The former is available in three sizes (standard dressings nos. 3, 4 and 5), and the dressing stretches across the shorter width of the fabric pad. The dressing is positioned on the skin surface so that the centre of the fabric pad is directly over the wound. The pad may be impregnated with a range of antiseptics (e.g. chlorhexidine hydrochloride or domiphen bromide) and dyed yellow. This is not always helpful, as it may cause irritation. The permeable plastic wound dressing is of a similar design, with the self-adhesive backing being perforated to allow the passage of water vapour and gases.

Semipermeable adhesive dressings are similarly constructed. However, the backing is not perforated but semipermeable and waterproof. It allows water vapour and gases to pass from the wound surface to the external environment, but prevents the movement of moisture in the opposite direction.

Occlusive adhesive dressings prevent the transference of water vapour and gases from the wound surface, but also minimise the inward transmission of microorganisms and dust. They may also prevent the spread of contamination from an infected wound to the surrounding area. They have a limited use for minor wounds only.

Adhesive dressing pads

Adhesive dressing pads (Table 5.1) consist of an absorbent pad which may be completely or partly surrounded by an adhesive plaster. Before use, the wound-facing surface is protected by a removable plastic-coated film. These products include many of the items described as 'plasters'. They are used in minor trauma as they minimise penetration of the wound by bacteria, but the absorbent pad is usually of only limited absorbency. Frequent changing may be required if the wound continues to suppurate, and this can damage the surrounding healthy epithelium.

Elastic adhesive dressing consists of an absorbent pad attached to an extension plaster coated with zinc oxide adhesive. It may be supplied as a wound dressing or as a strip dressing and can be used as a protective covering for many types of wound.

Perforated plastic wound dressing is similar to the elastic adhesive dressing. However, the adhesive dressing is a perforated plastic self-adhesive plaster which is permeable to water vapour and oxygen. An occlusive, waterproof version prevents the outward transmission of infection and the inward transmission of bacteria or dirt. The waterproof microporous plastic dressing can promote healing by allowing the

Table 5.1 Summary of the characteristics of adhesive dressing pads

Dressing	Waterproof	Water vapour permeable
Elastic dressing	No	Yes
Perforated plastic wound dressing	No	Yes
Waterproof plastic wound dressing	Yes	No
Waterproof microporous plastic wound dressing	Yes	Yes

passage of water vapour from the wound while maintaining a water-proof environment.

Bandages

Bandages can be classified for use as dressing retention materials, for support and for compression, according to their structure and predicted performance.

Retention bandages

Retention bandages can keep absorbent dressings in place or be used on their own to provide support for minor sprains and strains.

Non-extensible retention bandages include open-wove bandage, which is made of cotton or cotton and viscose, and triangular calico bandage, which is of greater strength and durability and can be used as a sling or a stump bandage. Domette bandage also contains wool and may be useful in dressing wounds where warmth is required. These bandages now have an extremely limited role as they have largely been replaced by more conformable products.

Retention bandages may also be made of stretch fabrics. Cotton conforming bandage is a two-way extensible bandage whose shape can be easily adapted to cover difficult sites of application. The elasticity can also provide support and keep an underlying wound management product in place. The warp threads in a polyamide and cellulose contour bandage are composed of crimped polyamide, which gives the bandage a longer life than a crepe bandage (see below). Tubular bandages may be made of gauze, stockinette (in which a cotton/viscose yarn is interspersed with a rubber thread) or cotton. Most are available in a range of sizes to cover a discrete area (e.g. hand, limb or body). An applicator may be supplied to position the bandage (e.g. over a limb or finger), and tubular bandages have the advantage over crepe bandages that an untrained person can apply them to produce an even distribution of pressure.

Support and compression bandages

Support and compression bandages commonly consist of fibres which stretch only along the length of the bandage. One-way stretch imparts support and pressure to the bandaged area and the degree of support varies according to the material of composition. Products are available whose use varies from minor conditions (e.g. mild strains and sprains) through to the firm support required after the removal of plaster. Support and compression bandages can also be classified as non-adhesive and adhesive.

Non-adhesive support and compression bandages (e.g. crepe bandage, cotton crepe bandage and cotton stretch bandage) are appropriate when light support is required. A crepe bandage contains wool and can provide warmth and insulation on exposed surfaces. It also has the advantage that elasticity lost during use may be at least partially restored by washing the bandage in warm soapy water. Medium support may be obtained through the use of cotton and rubber elastic bandage and heavy cotton and rubber elastic bandage. Patients may use cotton and rubber elastic bandage over long periods, and the heavy-duty version may retain its support properties even after several washings. A foot-loop may be present to assist in the correct positioning of the bandage on the limb.

The greatest degree of support in a non-adhesive support and compression bandage may be obtained by the use of an elastic web bandage. This has a distinctive blue line along its complete length and may be supplied with or without a foot-loop. The blue line provides a visual guide to the overlap required in application of the bandage. The bandage can be cut to any length and washed without loss of elasticity. A red-line version, which is heavier and gives even greater support, is also available.

Adhesive support and compression bandages may be self-adhesive or diachylon. Elastic adhesive bandage consists of an elastic cloth which may be completely spread with an adhesive (e.g. zinc oxide elastic self-adhesive bandage) or partially spread (e.g. half-spread zinc oxide elastic self-adhesive bandage). These bandages are used to provide support and compression (e.g. to swollen or sprained joints, leg ulcers and varicose veins). They are also commonly used to secure other appliances and wound management products. For application to large areas or to deep wounds a perforated version may be preferable (e.g. ventilated elastic adhesive bandage). Patients who are hypersensitive to rubber or zinc oxide can use titanium dioxide elastic adhesive bandage, which has the advantages over the zinc oxide self-adhesive bandages of less weight and enhanced porosity.

Diachylon bandages may be applied to skin (preferably shaved) by warming to activate the adhesive. The bandage may be occlusive (diachylon elastic adhesive bandage) or porous (ventilated diachylon elastic adhesive bandage). The absence of zinc oxide or rubber allows their use in sensitive patients.

One further product that may be considered to be self-adhesive but which does not have an adhesive coating is the cohesive extensible bandage. This bandage clings to itself, preventing slippage during use. It should not be used if arterial disease is suspected.

Medicated bandages

Medicated bandages combine the benefits of a cotton dressing with the use of an agent to reduce inflammation or promote healing, or both. A bandage can be kept in place for three to seven days. Particular care must be taken, however, to ensure that the patient does not react adversely to the incorporated agent. A wide range of medicaments can be incorporated into a bandage (e.g. zinc oxide, coal tar, ichthammol, calamine and clioquinol). Medicated bandages are used primarily in eczema, varicose veins, oedema and thrombophlebitis. When the bandage is put on the leg, the foot should be raised to improve venous drainage, and application should begin at the point nearest the toes.

A medicated stocking formed from rayon and covered with an ointment containing zinc oxide is also available for use with chronic leg ulcers. It may be used under appropriate compression hosiery when treating chronic venous insufficiency.

Multilayer compression bandaging

The application of uniform compression across the contours of the leg is the rationale behind the four-layer bandage system used to treat chronic leg ulcers, post-thrombotic venous insufficiency and gross oedema. The 'kits' available comprise a wound contact layer covered by a subcompression wadding bandage, a light compression bandage, and a fourth layer which may be selected to provide greater or lesser compression, depending on the degree of oedema present in the limb.

Wound dressing pads

Wound dressing pads consist of an absorbent pad enclosed in a sleeve of woven or non-woven fabric. The pad rapidly absorbs fluid and is therefore ideal for a grossly suppurating wound. It should not be used, however, if there is a risk of the wound drying out and the dressing sticking to the site of the trauma. A wound dressing pad can be retained in place by surgical adhesive tape or by a bandage.

The absorbent properties of wound dressing pads are due to the presence of knitted viscose, absorbent cotton and viscose, or absorbent cotton and crepe cellulose. The absorbent pad may be sleeved in a material which has been coated (e.g. with silicone, polyethylene, or polypropylene) to prevent adherence to the wound.

The most commonly used example of a wound dressing pad is the perforated film absorbent (PFA) dressing. This consists of a dry, non-adherent absorbent pad attached to gauze. The wound-contact surface is coated with a polyethylene film which is perforated to allow the passage of exudate into the pad. It is a flexible dressing, available in a range of sizes, and is ideally suited for awkwardly located wounds. Activated charcoal may be included in the sleeve layer. The deodorising action of the charcoal is especially useful for wounds which are infected and malodorous.

Tulle dressings

Tulle dressings (*tulle gras* = 'greased net') are non-adherent wound-contact dressings consisting of an open-weave fabric impregnated with white or yellow soft paraffin, but not so much as to produce a totally occlusive dressing. The dressing may be non-medicated (e.g. paraffin gauze dressing) or medicated (e.g. with chlorhexidine, framycetin, sodium fusidate or povidone-iodine).

Paraffin gauze dressing is used primarily for the treatment of burns, but it may also be useful as a 'barrier' dressing to prevent an outer, highly absorbent dressing from sticking to a wound. It has also been used as a packing material in decubitus ulceration and as an aid to the handling of skin grafts.

Chlorhexidine is an antiseptic with activity against many Gram-positive organisms, some Gram-negative bacteria, and fungi. It is relatively non-toxic and can be safely applied to large tracts of body surfaces (e.g. in excess of 10% of the body area).

Framycetin sulphate 1% is a broad-spectrum aminoglycoside antibiotic almost identical to neomycin. It may be used in a wide range of infected wounds (e.g. burns and scalds, skin grafts and stoma-induced skin problems). Although there is normally minimal systemic absorption of the antibiotic, the application of the dressing to large tracts of skin (> 30% body area) in which the epidermal barrier layers have been lost may lead to the characteristic ototoxicity of aminoglycosides.

Sodium fusidate gauze dressing contains sodium fusidate 2% ointment. It can be used in the treatment of wounds infected with Gram-positive organisms, particularly staphylococcal infections. Unlike other tulle dressings, it may not require the outer application of an absorbent dressing. It should also not be applied around or near the eye because of the risk of conjunctival irritation.

A non-adherent dressing containing povidone-iodine may be used to prevent the development of infection, particularly in burns. However, its activity is less than that of chlorhexidine because the antiseptic is inactivated by exudate from the wound.

Standard dressings

A list of standard dressings is given in Table 5.2. Most are obsolete and their use is not recommended because they interact with wounds by releasing fibres into the wound. These act as foreign bodies, thereby prolonging the inflammation phase of the healing process.

Surgical adhesive tapes

The classification of surgical adhesive tapes depends on the properties of the materials of construction. The backing material may be woven, non-woven or plastic. The adhesive may produce a tape which is permeable, allowing the passage of oxygen, water and bacteria; semipermeable, allowing the passage of oxygen and water vapour only; or occlusive. The choice of tape depends on the requirements for use and the type of skin surface to which it is to be applied. Common uses of surgical adhesive tape include:

- keeping intravenous infusion lines and urinary catheters in position;
- securing a dressing;
- restricting movement after orthopaedic surgery.

Permeable surgical adhesive tapes may comprise a woven backing fabric and are available with a range of adhesives. Adhesives containing zinc oxide are available on non-extensible (zinc oxide surgical adhesive) or extensible (elastic surgical adhesive) tapes. However, sensitivity to the adhesive may frequently arise and these tapes should not be used for prolonged periods. An alternative which may be used for extended periods is a woven tape with a polymeric adhesive (permeable woven surgical synthetic adhesive tape).

Non-woven synthetic materials are also used as the tape backing material. They are often preferable to woven fibres as their application permits the transmission of water vapour and oxygen while minimising the damage to healthy skin. Permeable non-woven surgical synthetic adhesive tape possesses less inherent strength than woven tape, but has

Table 5.2 Standard dressings

Number	Description
2	Fomentation dressing: consists of a polyethylene film and sterile lint, cotton wool and an open-weave bandage. Application is with magnesium sulphate paste or kaolin poultice as a fomentation dressing, or after the lint has been soaked as a wet dressing. Drying out is prevented by covering the dressing with the polyethylene film
3	Elastic adhesive wound dressing (pad size 20 x 25 mm)
4	Elastic wound dressing (pad size 10 or 30 × 50 mm)
5	Elastic wound dressing (pad size 35 × 60 mm): a central pad of lint (which may be impregnated with antiseptic) wrapped in muslin is fixed to an adhesive elastic plaster
6	Now replaced by self-adhesive dressing pads
7	Plain lint finger dressing: consists of a tube of lint inside an open-weave bandage. It may also be used on toes
8	Plain lint dressing (pad size 75 × 100 mm)
9	Plain lint dressing (pad size 100 × 150 mm): a three-layered dressing, comprising an inner lint surface, a pad of cotton wool and an outer open-weave bandage
10	Medicated lint finger dressing: similar to standard dressing no. 7, but with the lint impregnated with an antiseptic
11	Medicated lint dressing (pad size 75 × 100 mm)
12	Medicated lint dressing (pad size 100 × 150 mm): similar to standard dressings nos. 8 and 9, but with the lint impregnated with an antiseptic
13	Plain wound dressing (pad size 75 × 100 mm)
14	Plain wound dressing (pad size 100 × 150 mm)
15	Plain wound dressing (pad size 150 × 200 mm): consists of cotton wool enclosed in a gauze sleeve and attached to an open-weave bandage
16	Eye pad with bandage

the advantages of easy removal and handling. Greater strength may be obtained by the use of a 'ladder' technique of application (Figure 5.4).

Plastic film tapes may be perforated (permeable) or non-perforated (occlusive). They may be used to cover sites of infection while allowing the continued passage of oxygen and water vapour (e.g. permeable plastic surgical adhesive tape), or to cover sites where total exclusion of water and water vapour is required (e.g. impermeable plastic surgical synthetic adhesive tape and impermeable plastic surgical adhesive tape).

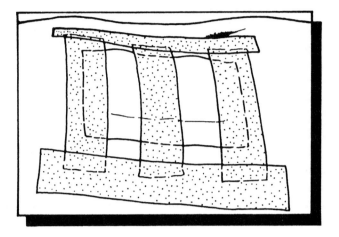

Figure 5.4 The 'ladder' technique for application of surgical adhesive tapes over larger dressings.

Modern wound management products

Recent innovations in wound management have been possible because of the greater understanding of the mechanism of wound healing and developments in polymer science. The characteristics of a product required for optimum wound healing can now be rationally selected, in stark contrast to the former empirical choice of agent. A range of products is available which have shown significant improvements in wound management over 'traditional' products.

The use of antiseptics is still common in the cleansing process associated with wound healing. This practice is not recommended, however, as it has been demonstrated that agents such as hypochlorites (contained, for example, in Eusol) interfere with the synthesis of new collagen and the budding of new capillaries.

A new range of debriding agents is now available which remove bacteria and dead cells and promote the formation of new granulation tissue. The presence of a defined structure in these new wound management products allows the cleansing process to be regulated, permitting effective removal of exudate but preventing drying-out of the wound.

Vapour-permeable adhesive film dressings

Film dressings are thin but very resilient semipermeable membranes formed of elastomeric copolymer, whose wound-contact surface is evenly coated with a synthetic adhesive. The film is impermeable to the inward passage of bacteria and water, but water vapour can escape from the wound surface. In the treatment of burns, less water vapour passes through the film than is lost from the traumatised skin surface, and a moist environment is therefore maintained at the wound surface. A significant advantage is the transparency of the film, which allows healing to be monitored without disturbing the wound site.

Preparation of the skin before the film dressing is applied is important. If the skin is wet or greasy, the film will not stay in place. The skin can be degreased with an alcohol swab. The presence of hair at the site of application may also reduce adhesion.

Film dressings are used in the treatment of a wide range of conditions, including pressure ulcers, burns, abrasions and donor sites. They can also be used to prevent the degradation of the skin surface caused, for example, by the close proximity of leg urine-drainage bags, and to keep infusion lines in position. Recently, film dressings have been introduced that are impregnated with an antibacterial (silver) for the management of infected wounds or a deodoriser (charcoal) for malodorous wounds.

The method of applying film dressings varies according to the manufacturer. It may require demonstration to patients before they gain sufficient confidence to apply the dressing themselves.

Polymeric foam dressings

Polymeric foam dressings are a diverse group of products with a wide range of properties. The first to be developed was a partially expanded, modified polyurethane foam. It comprised a lower layer of open cells and an upper hydrophilic surface with closed impermeable layers which reduced the loss of water vapour and prevented the passage of absorbed fluid. Polymeric foam dressings are useful for filling cavities as they assume the shape of the wound, exert pressure, and absorb exudate within the wound to stimulate the granulation process of wound healing. They may also be cut to the shape of the wound, and possess significant advantages over traditional wound-filling products (e.g. cellulose wadding or gauze). The dressings are available as sheets and as *in situ*-formed foams. They have a non-adherent wound-contact surface and are also available as adhesive island dressings and cavity fillers. They are available with or without an integral charcoal cloth to assist in the deodorisation of malodorous wounds, and in a wide range of sizes. The absorbent dressings can be used for wounds with moderate to heavy exudation, and are also recommended for the management of dry sutured wounds, minor lacerations, early pressure ulcers and venous ulcers.

These materials also demonstrate the greatest variability between products. The wound-contact layer is often heat treated, providing a smooth surface which absorbs fluids by capillarity. Creating a foam of the polymer creates small, open cells which are able to hold fluids; the cell size may be controlled during the foam-producing process. The sheet dressings are primarily polyurethane foams whose absorbency and water vapour permeability are varied either by a physical modification to the foam or by combining the foam with an additional sheet component. Their structure and softness also provide a cushion to protect and contribute to thermal insulation of the wound. They also may be tailored for particular applications (e.g. tracheostomy dressing) without particle loss to the wound and with the retention of their conformable characteristics. Non-adhesive foams require a secondary dressing.

Absorption of serous exudate is limited to the wound/dressing interface. The absorptive capacity of the hydrophobic portion can be exceeded in a high-exudate wound and, although moisture vapour transmission occurs through the dressing, frequent changes may be required until the exudate level diminishes. The use of a secondary absorbent pad will solve the problem of excess exudate while retaining the non-adherence, bacterial impermeability and gas and water vapour permeability functions, as well as the cushioning and thermal insulation properties of the foam.

When used as a primary dressing, the foam expands when wet and conforms to the contours of the wound, producing an environmental chamber with entrapped solutes and cell debris. It is claimed that this function enhances the inflammatory response of the wound and subsequently stimulates the production of granulation tissue and neovascularisation. These polyurethane membranes are recommended specifically for the management of stasis ulcers when used with a superimposed absorbent pad and graduated pressure applied either by stretch bandages or elasticated stockings.

A foam dressing with the prime function of absorbency has been designed for the management of burns. It consists of a highly absorbent hydrophilic polyurethane foam backed with a moisture-permeable polyurethane membrane and bonded to an apertured polyurethane net on the wound-contact face. It is capable of absorbing and retaining large volumes of fluid even under pressure. The backing is permeable to water vapour but impermeable to water. As the exudate level decreases, the matrix retains moisture and prevents the drying of the wound. The apertured polyurethane net interface reduces adherence to the wound surface. Although they are recommended primarily for burns, these dressings have been used successfully on other exuding lesions.

Low absorptive-capacity primary foam dressings have been produced from a carboxylated styrene butadiene rubber latex foam. The foam is bonded to a non-woven fabric coated with a polyethylene film which has been vacuum ruptured. The basic foam is naturally hydrophobic and a surface active agent is incorporated to facilitate the uptake of wound exudate. The polyethylene foam layer is particularly effective in preventing adherence, and the dressing is recommended for minor wounds and abrasions in which exudate levels are low and adherence a major hazard at dressing change.

In situ *foam*

One of the major problems in wound management is the treatment of large cavity wounds produced either postoperatively (e.g. a pilonidal sinus) or by trauma (e.g. pressure ulceration). It is necessary to occlude the cavity by packing to absorb excess exudate and to stimulate the production of granulation tissue, neovascularisation and collagen deposition.

The traditional procedure is to pack the cavity with variously impregnated ribbon gauze. The subsequent removal of such a dressing is difficult: the associated pain and stress may require low-level anaesthesia and theatre management.

An *in situ*-formed foam was originally designed by Dow Corning and found to be clinically superior to the ribbon gauze. It comprised a two-part foam composed of a filled polydimethylsiloxane base and a stannous octonate catalyst. (The catalyst is no longer used due to possible toxicity problems.) The two components are mixed together immediately prior to use. The reaction is slightly exothermic: over a period of two to three minutes the dressing expands to approximately four times its original volume and sets to a soft spongy foam that conforms accurately to the contours of the wound cavity. The stent is normally removed twice daily, soaked in a mild antiseptic (0.5% aqueous chlorhexidine) rinsed in cold running water, squeezed dry, and replaced. A new dressing is formed after a week or more to match the reduction in size of the cavity. The foam does not adhere to granulation tissue. It maintains free drainage around the wound and has a low but significant absorptive capacity at the dressing surface. It has been indicated for the management of pilonidal sinus, hidradenitis suppurativa, perianal and perineal wounds, and in the management of dehisced abdominal wounds.

Hydropolymer

This material looks like a foam but is described as a foamed gel formed from polyurethane. The material expands into the contours of the wound as it absorbs fluid. It is used in an island configuration with an adhesive portion which is unique, and has the ability to readhere once lifted, enabling manipulation of the product for fit or assessment of the wound without dressing change. The hydropolymer acts as a wick, drawing fluid into the upper layers of the dressing, where it passes through the backing. Its use is recommended for dynamic fluid management for heavily exuding wounds, or when extended periods between dressing changes are desirable.

Particulate and fibrous polymers

This group of dressings includes synthetic, semisynthetic and naturally occurring products comprising a range of polysaccharide materials.

Xerogels

Xerogel dressings may be regarded as a subgroup of products within the larger group of polysaccharide dressings. The latter contains the traditional cellulose dressing products (e.g. gauze and absorbent cotton). Products which consist of dextranomer beads, dehydrated hydrogels of the agar/acrylamide group, calcium alginate fibres, and dehydrated granulated Graft T starch polymers are identified specifically as xerogels, the material remaining after the removal of most or all of the water from a hydrogel (or the disperse phase from any type of simple gel). These materials therefore have no water in their formulation, but swell to form a gel when in contact with aqueous solutions.

Particulate polymers

Dextranomer is a polymer of the polysaccharide dextran, a naturally derived polymer of glucose produced by cultures of a microorganism, *Leuconostoc mesenteroides*. The gel is formed when the dextran molecules comprising the disperse phase of the hydrocolloid are cross-linked by a chemical process utilising epichlorhydrin and sodium hydroxide. Dextranomer is available as beads or paste. The material requires a secondary dressing.

The hydrophilic beads absorb the aqueous component of wound exudate and dissolved materials, ranging from inorganic salts to low molecular weight proteins. Microorganisms are removed from the wound by the capillary action between the beads, a function which is absent from the paste formulation. The paste formulation demonstrates a markedly better absorbent capacity for malodorous elements and pain-producing compounds released during the inflammatory response.

Dextranomer is used primarily as a debriding agent on sloughy and exuding wounds, whether clean or infected, and on small-area burns where the objective is to produce a clean tissue bed for the production of granulating tissue. It should not be used beyond this phase of healing, as its continued application will impair epithelialisation. Dextranomer is not biodegradable, and both granules and paste must be carefully removed with normal saline before drying to avoid particulate residues and the subsequent development of granulomas.

Its use on exudating necrotic injuries (e.g. leg ulcers) has proved beneficial, and it is an acceptable substitute for surgical or enzymatic debridement. The granules are contraindicated in drying wounds.

Fibrous polymers

Alginate dressings are composed of alginic acid, which is a polyuronic acid composed of residues of D-mannuronic acid and L-glucuronic acid. It is obtained chiefly from algae belonging to the Phaeophyceae, mainly species of *Laminaria*.

Calcium alginate dressings are flat, non-woven pads of either calcium sodium alginate fibre or solely calcium alginate fibre. The alginate wound-contact layer may be bonded to a secondary absorbent viscose pad. Alginate hanks are also available, and packing and ribbon can be used for deeper cavity wounds and sinuses. Alginates have been shown to be effective in the management of injuries where there has been substantial tissue loss. Non-adhesive formulations require a secondary dressing.

Gel formation is via ion exchange. A biodegradable gel is formed when the fibre is in contact with exudate; calcium contributes to the clotting mechanism. The gel may be firm or soft, depending upon the proportions of calcium and sodium in the fibre. It is removed with saline.

The isomeric acids are present in varying proportions, depending on the seaweed source. Calcium alginate is capable of gel formation. The glucuronic acid forms an association with calcium, providing the stimulus to produce the continuous disperse phase of a hydrogel. Calcium ions and a phospholipid surface promote the activation of prothrombin in the clotting cascade. Calcium alginate products are used as the source of these ions to arrest bleeding, both in superficial injuries and as an absorbable haemostat in surgery. The rate of biodegradation is related to the proportions of sodium and calcium in the preparation.

The 'wet' integrity of the dressing, which facilitates its removal from the wound, may be improved by incorporating fibres of greater strength (e.g. viscose (rayon) staple fibre) or fibres which interact with the alginate fibres when wet (e.g. chitosan staple fibres).

The primary haemostatic use of calcium alginate is in the packing of sinuses, fistulae and bleeding tooth sockets. The alginate dressings have recently become widely used as a soluble wound packing for a number of additional wound types. They are useful non-adherents for lacerations and abrasions, and are effective in the management of hyper-granulation tissue (proud flesh), interdigital maceration and heloma molle. Their hospital and community uses include intractable skin ulcers and pressure sores, in which they would appear to accelerate healing, and the successful management of diabetic ulcers, venous ulcers, burns and infected surgical wounds.

Alginates have proved useful debriding agents. When applied to these injury types the alginate must be covered by a secondary dressing of foam or film. Some proprietary products bond calcium alginate to a secondary backing (e.g. an absorbent viscose pad or semipermeable adhesive foam) to produce an island dressing.

Hydrogels

Hydrogels (water polymer gels) are modified cross-linked polymeric formulations. They form three-dimensional networks of hydrophilic polymers from materials such as gelatin, polysaccharides, cross-linked polyacrylamide polymers, polyelectrolyte complexes, and polymers or copolymers derived from methacrylate esters. These interact with aqueous solutions by swelling to an equilibrium value and retain a significant proportion of water within their structure. They are insoluble in water. Hydrogels are available as a dry or hydrated sheet or as a hydrated gel in sachets. When hydrated they contain up to 96% water and have additional, high absorption properties.

Their high moisture content maintains a desirable moist interface which facilitates cell migration and prevents dressing adherence. Water can be transmitted through the saturated gel; the unsaturated gel has a water vapour permeability comparable with that of vapour-permeable membranes.

The absorption, transmission and permeability performance result in the maintenance of a moist wound with a continuous moisture flux across the dressing and a sorption gradient which assists in the removal of toxic components from the wound area. The high moisture content allows dissolved oxygen permeability, the degree of which varies between products. This allows the continuation of aerobic function at the wound/dressing interface and benefits both epithelialisation and bacterial growth. It has been observed that the use of a hydrogel frequently results in a marked reduction in pain response in patients. It has been suggested that the high humidity protects the exposed neurons from dehydration and also produces beneficial changes in pH. A secondary effect which may contribute to this response is the property of the gels to immediately cool the wound surface and maintain a lower temperature for up to six hours. This lowering of temperature may reduce the inflammatory response.

Sheet hydrogels comprise three-dimensional networks of cross-linked hydrophilic polymers (polyethylene oxide, polyacrylamides, polyvinylpyrrolidone, carboxymethylcellulose, modified corn starch). Their formulation may incorporate up to 96% bound water, but they are insoluble in water and interact by three-dimensional swelling with aqueous solutions. The polymer physically entraps water to form a solid sheet. This may make the sheet feel moist, but compression will not release any water. They have a thermal capacity which provides initial cooling to the wound surface. A secondary dressing is required.

Recommended uses include the management of donor sites and superficial operation sites, burns, other painful wounds, and dermatitic skin where the avoidance of topical agents is indicated. In chronic ulcers they are used to encourage granulation and the formation of cellular tissue.

Amorphous hydrogels may have ingredients (e.g. alginate, collagen, or complex carbohydrates) in addition to water and a polymer. They are similar in composition to sheet hydrogels but the polymer has not been cross-linked. These amorphous preparations do not have the cooling properties of the sheet dressings and a secondary dressing is required. Recommended uses include hydration of dry, sloughy or necrotic wounds and autolytic debridement.

Hydrocolloids

Hydrocolloid dressings consist of composite products based on naturally occurring hydrophilic polymers. Generally these dressings are flexible, highly absorbent, occlusive or semiocclusive adhesive pads formulated from biocompatible hydrophilic polymers (e.g. sodium carboxymethylcellulose, hydroxyethylcellulose pectins and gelatin) incorporated into a hydrophobic adhesive. The dressings may be backed by a polymeric film and contoured to fit difficult areas. Hydrocolloids are also available as granules, pastes, powders or gels of similar formulation, allowing a continuous 'fill' for cavity wounds. The pads do not require a secondary dressing.

Other hydrocolloid dressings are also available, consisting of sodium carboxymethylcellulose alone or combined with karaya gum.

The adhesive property of hydrocolloids gives an initial adhesion higher than some surgical adhesive tapes. After application the absorption of transepidermal water vapour modifies the adhesive flow to maintain a high tack performance throughout use. *In situ*, the dressings provide a gas- and moisture-proof environment strongly attached to the area surrounding the wound and offering protection against contamination (e.g. from incontinence). In the wound-contact area the exudate is absorbed to form a gel that swells in a linear fashion, with a higher moisture retention at the contact surface (Figure 5.5). This results in an expansion of the gel into the wound cavity, with continued support and increasing pressure from the remainder of the elastomeric dressing. The larger the volume of exudate, the greater the expansion into the cavity up to the limitation imposed by the availability of the gel. The advantage of this system is that it applies a firm pressure to the floor of a deep ulcer, a basic surgical maxim for the production of healthy granulating tissue. It is this function that contributes to its recommended usage for venous ulcers.

The formed 'colloidal' gel also produces a sorption gradient for soluble components within the serous exudate and allows the removal of toxic compounds derived from bacterial or cellular destruction. The moist gel is soft and conforms to the wound contours. When the dressing is removed, the gel remains in the wound and can be washed away with saline. During use the dressing in contact with the wound liquefies to produce a pus-like liquid with a somewhat strong odour. The hydrocolloids are suitable for desloughing and for light- to medium-exuding wounds, but are contraindicated if an anaerobic infection is present. Recommended uses for these dressings include pressure ulcers, minor

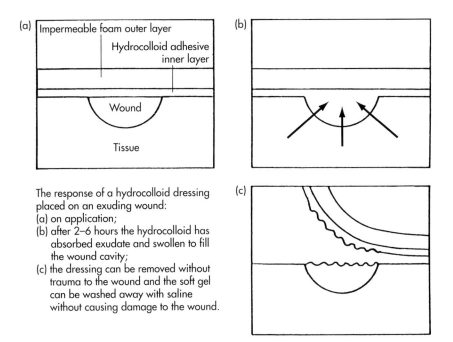

(a) Impermeable foam outer layer

Hydrocolloid adhesive inner layer

Wound

Tissue

The response of a hydrocolloid dressing placed on an exuding wound:
(a) on application;
(b) after 2–6 hours the hydrocolloid has absorbed exudate and swollen to fill the wound cavity;
(c) the dressing can be removed without trauma to the wound and the soft gel can be washed away with saline without causing damage to the wound.

Figure 5.5 The action of a hydrocolloid dressing.

burns, granulating wounds, wounds exhibiting slough or necrotic tissue, and wounds with moderate exudate.

Superabsorbents

These are hydrocolloidal compounds that have a high absorbent capacity and entrap exudate so that it cannot be squeezed out once absorbed. One product incorporates this material into an island pad which is covered by a non-woven absorbent and surrounded by an extra-thin hydrocolloid as the adhesive portion. The covering acts as a transfer layer while its surface stays dry. They are recommended for use with heavily exuding ulcers.

Hydrofibres

Hydrofibres are fibres of carboxymethylcellulose formed into flat, non-woven pads that form a gel in contact with fluid. The absorbency rate and capacity are approximately three times those of calcium alginate. The resultant gel is similar to a sheet hydrogel and does not dry out. Therefore, there is no maceration of the skin surrounding the wound, but moisture is maintained in contact with the wound bed. The high absorbent capacity reduces the frequency of dressing changes. They are recommended for use with heavily exuding wounds or wounds requiring long-term dressing.

Biodressings

Biodressings are composed of materials almost exclusively derived from living tissue and are said to 'participate actively and beneficially in the biochemistry and cellular activity of wound healing'. They are classified into biological and biosynthetic dressings; biological dressings can be further subdivided into natural or cultured, depending on their origin. Their use requires expert assessment and manipulation.

Further reading

Cohen IK, Diegelmann RF, Lindblad WJ, eds. (1992). *Wound Healing: Biochemical and Clinical Aspects*. Philadelphia: WB Saunders.

Krasner DK, Kane D, eds (1997). *Chronic Wound Care: A Clinical Source for Healthcare Professionals*. Wayne, PA: Health Management Publications.

Peacock EE (1984). *Wound Repair*. Philadelphia: WB Saunders.

Thomas S (1990). *Wound Management and Dressings*. London: Pharmaceutical Press.

Yardley PA (1998). *A Brief History of Wound Healing*. Oxford: Oxford Clinical Communications.

6

Oxygen therapy

Derrick Garwood

Oxygen has been used therapeutically since the First World War to overcome low blood levels of the gas (hypoxaemia). Initially, the uncontrolled use of high-concentration oxygen chambers to treat lobar pneumonia led to side-effects (e.g. convulsions, lung damage, and occasionally death). Since the 1960s, however, it has been recognised that continuous low concentrations of oxygen can improve the quality and prolong the life of patients suffering from hypoxaemia and the consequent deficiency of oxygen in the tissues (tissue hypoxia).

Indications for oxygen therapy

Any condition that causes hypoxaemia can lead to tissue hypoxia, which produces symptoms that include confusion, excitement, headache, nausea, disorientation, and eventually unconsciousness.

Hypoxia may result from either an acute shortage of oxygen or from long-term pathology. Oxygen therapy can be used to treat acute disturbances of respiratory function (e.g. an asthma attack), but this chapter focuses on long-term oxygen therapy in conditions such as chronic bronchitis and emphysema.

Hypoxia may be classified as follows:

- Hypoxic hypoxia is characterised by inefficient blood oxygenation caused by obstruction of the air passages, or by any physical barrier that impedes the transference of oxygen into arterial blood (e.g. in emphysema and degenerative tissue damage). Acute hypoxic hypoxia leads to hyperventilation and increased carbon dioxide elimination. Chronic hypoxic hypoxia also generates increased numbers of circulating red blood cells (secondary polycythaemia) which, together with pulmonary hypertension, can result in right ventricular failure (cor pulmonale).
- Anaemic hypoxia results from a reduced oxygen-carrying capacity of red blood cells. This may be due to decreased haemoglobin

content or the presence of another agent which has preferentially bound to haemoglobin (e.g. carbon monoxide). Most cases of anaemic hypoxia produce only rare breathlessness at rest, but significant respiratory embarrassment on exercise.

- Ischaemic or stagnant hypoxia may occur locally, or generally if the circulation of blood slows. The most common causes are very low temperatures (which produce severe vasoconstriction), cardiac failure and peripheral circulatory failure.

- Histotoxic hypoxia commonly arises from poisoning, usually by cyanide or narcotic agents. The presence of the poison prevents oxygen being utilised by the tissues, even though blood gas levels may be normal.

'Pink puffers' and 'blue bloaters'

The degree of blood oxygenation and, by inference, the extent of tissue hypoxia can be assessed from the colour of the skin. Cyanosis gives a violet-blue tinge to the skin, as a result of high levels of reduced haemoglobin in the peripheral blood vessels. In chronic respiratory disease, cyanosis results from abnormal mixing of oxygenated and deoxygenated blood.

Breathlessness and hyperinflation of the chest produce the characteristic 'pink puffer', whose peripheral blood flow is very rapid and whose extremities are warm and highly coloured. These effects result from the compensatory mechanism of vasodilatation attempting to improve the circulation. The redness of the blood indicates only a mild degree of hypoxaemia, coupled to the nearly normal removal of carbon dioxide. The outward signs of the 'pink puffer' are seen predominantly in pulmonary emphysema. Patients are generally aged 60–70 years, thin, and present with little or no cough and only small amounts of sputum.

By comparison, the 'blue bloater' requires urgent action. Such patients are severely cyanosed and the venous pulse may be difficult to detect. Hypoxaemia is persistent. Attempts to improve the level of tissue oxygenation lead to secondary polycythaemia. Sputum production is considerable and the sputum is usually infected. A rattling cough persists caused by attempts to remove the sputum, whose presence produces an inspiratory wheeze and breathlessness. These signs and symptoms are usually the result of chronic bronchitis. In the later stages, oedema in the ankles and neck indicates deterioration towards right-sided heart failure caused by pulmonary hypertension. Not all patients present with breathlessness, but those who do may appear irritable and hostile.

Chronic bronchitis

Chronic bronchitis is defined as prolonged exposure to non-specific irritants which cause the production of excessive, viscous and frequently infected mucus, together with changes in pulmonary structure. In its early stages, blockage of the peripheral mucosa, rather than the central portions of the lungs, occurs. Consequently, the resistance to air-flow increases and greater physical effort is required for normal breathing.

Non-uniform mucus production leads to ventilation–perfusion mismatch and eventually hypoxaemia. The removal of waste carbon dioxide becomes less efficient, producing a compensatory increase in bicarbonate ion reabsorption by the kidneys to prevent metabolic acidosis.

Inflammation in the lungs reduces the number and functioning of cilia, further impairing the removal of mucus. The cough mechanism attempts to compensate for reduced ciliary action, but if the mucus is highly infected and deep breathing is not possible, this mechanism is severely compromised. Mucus remains deep-seated, infections frequently occur, and many patients contract bronchopneumonia.

The most common cause of chronic bronchitis is cigarette smoke. Irritants in the inhaled gases cause increased mucus production and damage the cilia. Constriction of the airways produced by smoking acts as a further obstacle to the removal of mucus. Other irritants that can have similar effects are inhaled dust or other forms of air pollution (e.g. asbestos particles). Such agents produce non-specific degenerative changes in lung function.

Patients who expose themselves to such irritants and are therefore susceptible to lung infections are particularly vulnerable during the cold winter months. Mucus lodged in the bronchi acts as a growth medium for invading microorganisms. Recurrent infections, compounded by hypoxaemia, lead to a general deterioration in health. Poor appetite, weight loss and general inactivity are common indicators of this condition, which frequently leads to premature death from bronchopneumonia, other serious respiratory infections or right-sided heart failure (cor pulmonale).

Emphysema

In this condition the reduced elasticity of lung tissue – usually the bronchioles – leads to dilatation of the alveoli. This may develop asymptomatically over a period of time, so that many patients do not seek medical advice until considerable tissue damage has occurred. Where the damage is limited to the terminal bronchioles, the condition is termed centrilobular emphysema; if the whole lobule is affected, the emphysema is described as panlobular.

Tissue damage causes oedema and eventually fibrosis. The reduced elasticity in the airways traps air in the lungs, particularly if there is excessive mucus secretion. As a result, the lungs and chest cavity become hyperinflated. Oedema also impairs gaseous exchange, producing breathlessness. However, unlike chronic bronchitis, cough and sputum do not usually contribute significantly to the clinical picture.

The body attempts to compensate for breathlessness in several ways. Pursed lips endeavour to increase the duration of expiration, prevent bronchiolar collapse, and decrease the likelihood of more air becoming trapped. Patients may also sit with their hands on their thighs to improve the action of the respiratory muscles. The chest becomes barrel-shaped and enlarged, and overall the body is thin and emaciated owing to loss of appetite.

The involvement of proteolytic enzymes in lung tissue damage has been suggested. It is believed that these enzymes normally eliminate debris from inhaled material and particles shed from the lung surface. Their activity is controlled by another enzyme, α_1-antitrypsin (αAT). In certain genetic disorders, and in the presence of irritants such as cigarette smoke, the activity of αAT decreases, leading to excessive proteolysis that causes widespread lung tissue damage.

Comparison of oxygen requirements and their fulfilment

Among many other modalities (e.g. stopping smoking, occupational therapy, physiotherapy) the provision of oxygen is an important treatment for hypoxia. The primary objective is to improve resting and exercise levels of blood oxygen; therapy is *not* intended to return blood levels to those of an individual with competent lung function. Oxygen must be regarded in the same manner as any other drug, because its incorrect use may produce harmful rather than beneficial effects.

Ideally, oxygen should be administered continuously at an inspired concentration appropriate to the degree of tissue hypoxia. Thoracic consultants usually assess patients' oxygen requirements by measuring the forced expiratory volume in one second (FEV_1). Arterial blood pressure measurements may also be correlated with blood haemoglobin levels.

In chronic conditions such as bronchitis and emphysema the oxygen concentration must normally be kept below 40%: low-dose continuous therapy typically utilises inspired concentrations of 24–30% at a flow rate of 2 L/min. Administration of this concentration for between 12 and 19 hours in every 24 has been shown to significantly reduce the mortality rate of these conditions. This treatment reduces erythrocyte mass and pulmonary arterial pressure, thereby decreasing the frequency of hospital admissions.

If oxygen therapy is continued throughout sleep, the risk of developing severe hypoxaemia, particularly during rapid eye movement (REM) sleep, is diminished. Such reductions in blood oxygen levels result from reduced ventilation and a nocturnal rise in pulmonary arterial pressure, and increase the risk of right-sided heart failure.

Oxygen is supplied to the patient from a storage or generating system via a delivery system. A storage or generating system may be an oxygen cylinder, an oxygen concentrator, or liquid oxygen. The delivery system is a mask, a nasal cannula/prongs, or a nasal catheter. Selection of the appropriate equipment is determined by the duration of therapy, the mobility of the patient and the quantity of oxygen required.

For low oxygen use (intermittent therapy, or for less than 8 hours per day), cylinders are the most appropriate. Although cylinder use implies a degree of immobility, systems can be installed which store cylinders in one room and pipe gas to outlets in other parts of the home. Small-capacity portable cylinders are also available for trips away from home.

For high oxygen use (more than eight hours per day) a concentrator is more cost-effective and takes up less room than the cylinders required to provide an equivalent volume of gas.

In some countries liquid oxygen may be administered from a portable device and this is particularly suitable for an ambulant patient.

Oxygen cylinders

In the UK, NHS form FP10 (GP10 in Scotland) allows a general practitioner to prescribe the following equipment: an oxygen cylinder, cylinder stand, domiciliary oxygen headset or regulator, and a face mask. This prescription may be dispensed by any community pharmacy authorised by the appropriate Health Authority (Health Board in Scotland) to provide domiciliary oxygen therapy services. Authorised oxygen contractors agree to fulfil a number of service requirements, including:

• To stock sufficient oxygen cylinders and equipment at the pharmacy to meet the anticipated demand

- To transport cylinders and equipment to and from patients' homes – this is essential because patients or their representatives may be physically unable to do so
- To set up the equipment in patients' homes and explain its use
- To provide a leaflet explaining the use, care, and safe storage of all items supplied
- To ensure that any representative acting on behalf of a patient is capable of transporting, erecting and operating the equipment
- To ensure that equipment loaned to patients is clearly marked with a label stating that it is the property of the pharmacy and must be returned in good condition if no longer required
- To arrange collection of all equipment if notified by the Health Authority (Health Board) that it is no longer required.

Pharmacies are not obliged to register as oxygen contractors. If a prescription for oxygen is presented at a pharmacy which is not registered, the pharmacist must give the names, addresses and telephone numbers of at least two registered pharmacies which are located near the patient's home.

Any pharmacy can apply to its local Health Authority (Health Board) to provide an oxygen therapy service. Applications are considered by the Local Pharmaceutical Committee (Area Pharmaceutical Committee in Scotland), whose recommendations are passed to the Health Authority (Health Board) to make the final decision on the basis of whether the proposed service is both necessary and desirable.

Payment under the NHS

Payment for providing an oxygen therapy service has two distinct components: one for the provision of oxygen, and the other for the pharmacist's professional services. Prescriptions for oxygen should be endorsed with the name of the oxygen set provided and the start date and quantity of cylinders supplied, and then submitted to the Prescription Pricing Authority each month along with all other NHS prescriptions. Payments for professional services, including delivery, rental fees for the equipment, and domiciliary visits, are claimed directly from the relevant Health Authority, using their individual claim forms.

Some Health Authorities (Health Boards) allocate an 'Authorised Holding' to each registered oxygen contractor. This is the number of oxygen headsets for which the Authority is prepared to pay a monthly rental fee and approve delivery charges, and includes a provision for spares. Other Authorities will only pay rental fees for headsets that are actually in use by patients.

If a pharmacy suffers a financial loss because equipment is lost or damaged by a patient, it should present a claim to the appropriate Health Authority, in accordance with that Authority's specific regulations.

Types of oxygen cylinder

Steel cylinders containing oxygen for use in the home are available in a range of sizes, including:

- 3400 L at 137 bar pressure (13 650 kPa)
- 1360 L at 137 bar pressure (13 650 kPa)
- 2122 L at 200 bar pressure (21 300 kPa) (these cylinders have an integral valve/regulator which prevents headsets rated for the lower pressure being used).

Oxygen cylinders are colour-coded, having a black body with a white shoulder. Their strong construction means that, even when empty, the 1360 L cylinder weighs 14.5 kg. This is an important consideration in delivery and collection. Each cylinder also has a tag stating the date of supply, the batch number, and the site at which it was filled.

In the UK, oxygen is normally supplied in standard 1360 L cylinders. Their use is now limited to low-demand patients, because one cylinder must be supplied each week for approximately every *hour* per day that oxygen is required at a flow rate of 2 L/min.

Prescriptions on form FP10 (GP10) for smaller (170 L and 340 L) oxygen cylinders are passed for payment in the same way as prescriptions for drugs (i.e. not as part of the oxygen therapy service). However, these smaller cylinders require a different headset from standard cylinders, and this cannot be provided under current NHS regulations. Therefore, unless a patient buys the appropriate headset, or has been provided with one by the hospital services, the pharmacist cannot supply these cylinders because the patient is unable to use them.

Portable oxygen cylinders (PD cylinders) containing 300 L of oxygen at a pressure of 137 bar can also be specified on FP10. These are not currently included in the *Drug Tariff* regulations, and therefore no delivery fee can be claimed. However, in England and Wales the Prescription Pricing Authority will reimburse contractors for the cost of the gas. The rental fee can also be reclaimed as 'out-of-pocket expenses' by attaching an explanatory note to the FP10. In Scotland, however, the PPD will not pay rental fees for PD cylinders.

Headsets

Compressed gas in the cylinder is reduced to a pressure of between 70 and 415 kPa by its passage through the headset (also termed sets, regulators or control heads) (Figure 6.1). The calibrated pressure gauge must have at least '¼', '½', and 'FULL' markings, and its reading correlates directly with the amount of gas remaining in the cylinder.

The passage of oxygen from the cylinder can be regulated by settings which correspond to flow-rates of 0, 2 and 4 L/min. These settings are controlled by a ratchet device, which may either be incorporated into the headset or separate (specifications 01A and 01B, respectively). The outlet from the headset is connected to the delivery tube by a male bayonet fitting (see Figure 6.1).

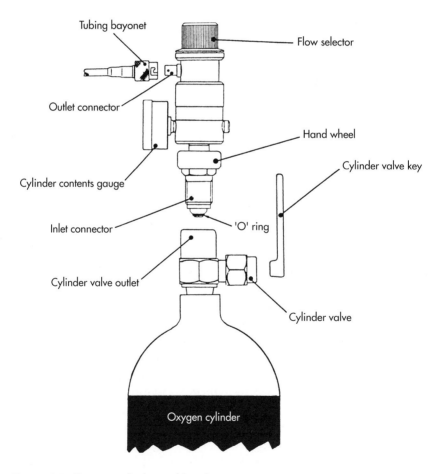

Figure 6.1 Oxygen cylinder and headset.

Standard cylinders utilise a separate lightweight headset which is supplied in a box complete with connecting tubing, a cylinder key or spanner, a mask, and instructions for use. The headset is connected to the cylinder by a bull-nose adaptor which must be only hand-tightened (patients should be warned against overtightening). A neoprene O-ring washer is used to create a gastight seal between the cylinder and the headset. Most leaks can be rectified by replacing the O-ring, but this operation should only be carried out by the pharmacist.

In order to simplify the operation of the equipment, some cylinders now incorporate an integral headset. This eliminates the need to connect the patient's headset to each new cylinder and reduces the likelihood of leaks.

Setting up the equipment

When a standard cylinder is delivered, the valve outlet is sealed by a plastic cap. This should be removed and the complete absence of dust confirmed by momentarily opening and immediately closing the valve using the key or spanner supplied, a process known as 'cracking' the valve. (Alternatively, some cylinders may have a simple handwheel which operates the valve.) It is also important to allow the cylinder to reach room temperature before use by the patient, especially if the cylinder is cold.

The headset is fitted and the cylinder valve gently opened. The pressure gauge on the headset should indicate that the cylinder is full. If, with the headset in the 'OFF' position the reading falls, either the seal is inadequate or the headset is faulty. An unsatisfactory seal may result from the O-ring washer having been placed incorrectly. Under no circumstances should oil or grease be used on the joint between cylinder and headset.

Patients should be told that the pressure gauge reading will gradually fall during use. They should also be reassured that, when the needle enters the red portion of the gauge, up to 25% of the oxygen remains, sufficient for two to three hours' use.

The contractor may consider that a cylinder stand is required to secure the cylinder and avoid the risk of accident to the patient. If so, then a stand may be provided on loan. However, the majority of Health Authorities will no longer pay for stand rental, and no payments are now allowed in Scotland.

Once the cylinder is empty the headset should be removed. Pressure within the headset may be released by closing the cylinder valve and setting the headset to the 'ON' position. The cylinder should then be stored to await collection and return to the supplier. Both empty and full cylinders should be kept in a dry, well-aired environment not subject to significant changes in temperature. They should preferably be stored upright on a cylinder stand or trolley. If this is not practicable, they should be laid horizontally on wooden shelves. Care must be taken to avoid damaging the cylinders in transit.

When delivering a cylinder with an integrated headset, it is only necessary to remove the cover from the outlet (on to which the mask and tubing fit) and 'crack' the valve. The patient may then begin using the cylinder as soon as it has reached room temperature.

Oxygen concentrators

Long-term, high-use oxygen therapy in the home may be provided by oxygen concentrators, which can be prescribed by a general practitioner on form FP10. These electrically powered machines extract oxygen from the atmosphere and deliver the concentrated gas directly to the patient (Figure 6.2). At present, UK pharmacies do not deal with prescriptions

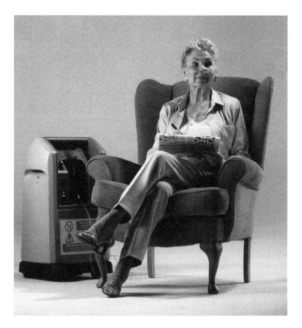

Figure 6.2 Patient receiving concentrator therapy (courtesy of BOC Vitalair, part of the BOC Group).

for oxygen concentrators. Instead, a single specialist supplier has been appointed to each regional group of Health Authorities.

Patients suitable for oxygen concentrator therapy are those with chronic obstructive airways disease and hypoxaemia (see above). Hypercapnia (abnormally high carbon dioxide levels in the blood) and oedema may also be present. Shorter-term but equally intensive use may be appropriate for patients in the final stages of other lung diseases (e.g. lung cancer, sarcoidosis, pneumoconiosis and alveolitis).

Once the initial outlay for a concentrator has been met, its running costs are approximately half that of cylinders for equivalent treatment. It is considered cost-effective to switch to a concentrator if the patient is using 21 cylinders or more per month.

Oxygen concentrators work on one of two principles:

- As a molecular sieve (Figure 6.3). Air is passed into a cylindrical sieve containing zeolite crystals, which adsorb nitrogen and hydrocarbons. The adsorption of oxygen is minimised by carefully timing the running cycle. The concentrated oxygen is removed to a storage tank and the inward airflow is then diverted to a second adsorbing sieve. Meanwhile, the first sieve is purged of nitrogen and other materials by the action of a vacuum, or by backflow of some of the stored oxygen. Theoretically, the sieves could last indefinitely; in practice, contamination with atmospheric moisture reduces their efficiency.

- As a semipermeable membrane. Oxygen is extracted from air by the selective passage of water vapour and oxygen through a semipermeable membrane. The device works by a vacuum action and therefore has fewer moving parts than the molecular sieve version.

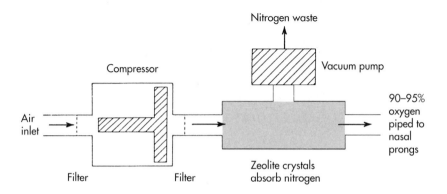

Figure 6.3 Oxygen concentrator – molecular sieve theory.

Most concentrators in the UK work on the molecular sieve principle and deliver approximately 90% pure oxygen. Technological improvements have led to a reduction in unit size, to about 70 cm high, 40 cm wide and 35 cm deep (Figure 6.4). Concentrators typically weigh about 20 kg and can be moved relatively easily. Correct positioning of the unit is extremely important. It must be:

• in a well-ventilated area with a good circulation of fresh air
• at least 30 cm from walls, curtains, furniture or other objects that could obstruct the air intake
• well away from any sources of heat or ignition (e.g. radiators and fireplaces)
• close enough to a power socket to prevent accidental unplugging.

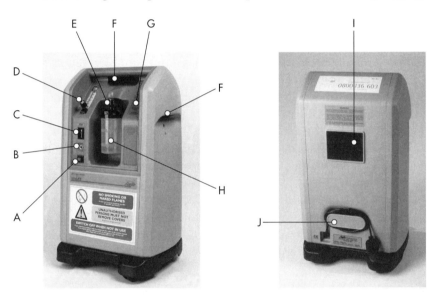

A   **On/off power switch**
B   **Circuit breaker reset button:** resets the unit after electrical overload shutdown
C   **Hour meter:** records the unit's total hours of operation
D   **Illuminated flowmeter/adjustment knob:** controls and indicates the oxygen flow in litres per minute (L/min).
E   **Oxygen outlet:** provides connections for a humidifier (if required), cannula or mask
F   **Top and side handles**
G   **Operating instructions**
H   **Humidifier**
I   **Air intake filter:** prevents dust and other airborne particles from entering the unit
J   **Power cord:** allows connection of unit into an electrical outlet

Figure 6.4 Main features of an oxygen concentrator (courtesy of BOC Vitalair, part of the BOC Group).

There are two installation options. The 'wheel-in' option allows the concentrator to be moved from room to room. Alternatively, it may be permanently located in one room or hallway and the oxygen piped to a number of outlets in other rooms, so that the patient can be mobile.

Most devices incorporate filter, pressure and valve alarms. The flowmeter on the front panel (see Figure 6.4) is manually set by the installer to the prescribed flow rate. Tamper-proof devices are available to prevent patients making their own adjustments. The duration of usage may be recorded by an internal clock (see Figure 6.4), to ensure patient compliance with the prescribed regimen and economic use of the apparatus.

The concentrator requires very little maintenance by the patient: typically, just a regular wiping of the surface with a damp cloth and washing of the air intake filter. Quarterly and annual services are carried out in the patient's home by an engineer sent by the specialist supplier. At these visits, the engineer also assesses the amount of electricity used by the concentrator, so that the patient can be reimbursed for electricity costs.

Concentrators are generally reliable, but in the event of a breakdown suppliers must respond to an emergency call-out within 10 hours. Most patients are not clinically at risk if their oxygen supply is interrupted for a few hours, but doctors may prescribe emergency back-up cylinders for those who are vulnerable. These are normally provided by the concentrator supplier.

Oxygen inspired by the patient may require humidification, particularly if the gas is administered by nasal catheter. Where this is the case, a humidifier is normally included on the FP10 (GP10) form prescribing the oxygen concentrator. The humidifier may connect directly to the concentrator (see Figure 6.4), or be a completely separate unit. It is important that the humidifier water chamber is filled to the correct level with fresh distilled water each day, and not allowed to run dry.

Liquid oxygen

Liquid oxygen systems (Figure 6.5) enable oxygen-dependent patients to enjoy freedom of movement both in the home and away from it. They are therefore most suitable for patients who are still in employment or fit enough to enjoy gentle outdoor activities. These systems cannot currently be provided by the National Health Service.

A typical system includes a 30 L reservoir cylinder of liquid oxygen, capable of delivering over 25 000 L of gas, located at the patient's home. There is also a portable 1.2 L cylinder which is filled from the reservoir

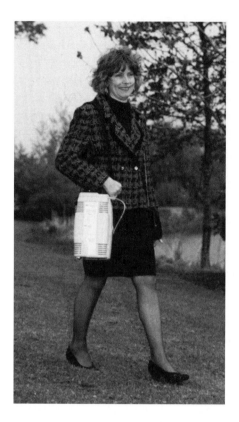

Figure 6.5 Using a portable liquid oxygen cylinder (courtesy of BOC Vitalair, part of the BOC Group).

to provide sufficient oxygen for a normal day's activity. Complete filling takes approximately one minute. The portable cylinder provides up to eight hours of oxygen gas at a flow rate of 2 L/min, but weighs less than 4 kg when full and can easily be carried by many patients using a shoulder strap. The flow control valve can be locked by the supplier to ensure that the prescribed flow rate is not exceeded.

Oxygen delivery systems

Masks

The traditional method of delivering medical gases is through a mask. Masks are relatively easy to use and precise concentrations of gas can be administered with constant-performance masks (see below). However, masks are occlusive and prevent normal speaking and eating. Patients may find them difficult to tolerate, particularly if a poor seal between face and mask causes an irritating draught over the face.

Two types of mask may be prescribed on form FP10 (GP10): constant performance and variable performance. If the type of mask is not specified, a constant-performance device should be provided.

Constant-performance (Venturi) masks

These masks provide an almost constant concentration of 28% oxygen in air, irrespective of the flow rate and the patient's breathing pattern. The most economical flow rate is 2 L/min, which corresponds to the 'MEDIUM' setting on the headset. The position of the mask on the face is less critical than with variable-performance masks. Unused and expired gases pass through outlets near the edge of the mask. These may help to keep the patient's face cool, but may also create a disturbing background noise.

Examples of constant-performance masks are the Intersurgical 010 Mask 28% and the Ventimask Mk IV 28%.

Variable-performance masks

These masks can supply a much higher concentration of oxygen and their use is restricted primarily to acute conditions (e.g. asthma, pulmonary oedema and pneumonia). To prevent a rapid rise in the concentration of inspired oxygen the patient must possess a good ventilatory drive. A flow rate of 2 L/min is recommended, and the concentration of inspired oxygen depends on:

- the rate of oxygen flow: as this increases, the inspired oxygen concentration increases
- the breathing pattern of the patient (e.g. tidal volume and rate of breathing)
- the amount of rebreathing permitted by the mask
- the position of the mask on the face.

Examples of variable-performance masks are the Intersurgical 005 Mask and the Venticaire Mask.

Each mask is provided for one patient only. Patients should be instructed to wipe the mask with a clean, dry cloth after use to remove any condensation. Masks should be replaced once they become cloudy or discoloured, which generally takes two to four months, depending on the level of use.

Nasal catheters and cannulae (prongs)

Patients receiving long-term oxygen therapy may not tolerate the prolonged intrusion on their lifestyle that wearing an oxygen mask can cause, preferring the less restrictive nasal catheter or nasal cannula. These devices allow normal speech and eating during therapy, but cannot currently be provided on form FP10. (In Scotland, the Intersurgical 1161 nasal cannula may be prescribed on form GP10.)

Nasopharyngeal catheters are usually restricted to hospital use because of the specialised insertion procedure and the need for the catheter to be switched to the alternative nostril every four to six hours. A further complication is the need for humidification by a gas-driven or ultrasonic nebuliser or water humidifier. This is necessary because, in normal breathing, the inspired air is warmed and collects moisture as it passes through the mouth and nose. The nasopharyngeal catheter bypasses this mechanism, making external humidification essential.

A nasal cannula is a disposable device consisting of two short, soft PVC prongs connected to hollow plastic tubing. The prongs project into the nostrils, and the plastic tubing is attached to a headset or oxygen concentrator. The device can be held in place by an elastic strap or a loop-like arrangement of tubing which passes behind the ears and is brought forward under the chin (Figure 6.6).

Humidification is generally considered unnecessary with nasal cannulae, because the moisture that accumulates during the passage of the gas into the lungs is normally sufficient to prevent irritation of the internal mucous membranes. However, wearing cannulae for long periods can cause drying of the nasal passages, soreness and encrustation. For susceptible patients, humidification is beneficial. If encrustation does develop, it can be removed by gently washing the nostrils two or three times a day.

Safety measures in the home

Oxygen itself is not flammable but it increases the rate of burning of any flammable substance. This effect is particularly pronounced when the concentration of oxygen rises above the 20% normally found in the atmosphere. Some materials that do not burn in air will burn in oxygen, and the accumulation of static electricity (which can generate sparks) is more likely to cause combustion in an oxygen-rich atmosphere.

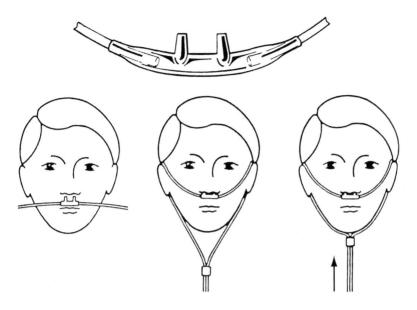

Figure 6.6 Nasal cannula.

To prevent accidents – especially fires – the following rules must be observed:

- No one must smoke in the vicinity of a patient receiving oxygen.
- Oil, grease or petroleum products must never be used on or near oxygen cylinders or concentrators, to prevent the risk of combustion.
- Patients must not use vapour rub or petroleum jelly, excessive amounts of skin lotion or face cream, or aerosol sprays while receiving oxygen.
- Patients must not receive oxygen close to a source of ignition (e.g. an open fire, paraffin or bottled gas heater, or gas stove).
- Patients should receive therapy away from sources of heat (e.g. radiators).
- The flow of oxygen should be turned off as soon as therapy is complete.
- Long lengths of tubing should be draped over hooks positioned above floor level, to prevent tripping or damage to the equipment.
- Care must be taken to ensure that tubing does not become kinked or occluded (e.g. by running a vacuum cleaner over it).

Liquid oxygen presents additional problems. Under no circumstances should patients transfer the liquefied gas into a portable canister other than the one provided: the very low temperature may cause other container materials to become brittle and crack. Patients should also be warned that if liquid oxygen comes into contact with the skin, severe burns will result. Should such an accident occur, the skin should be washed with plenty of water.

Further reading

Adams FV (1999). *The Breathing Disorders Sourcebook*. New York: Verulam Publishing.

Bellamy D, Booker R, Barnes G, Calverley P (1999). *Chronic Obstructive Pulmonary Disease in Primary Healthcare*. London: Class Publishing.

Haas F, Sperber Haas S (2000). *The Chronic Bronchitis and Emphysema Handbook*. Chichester: John Wiley.

Jenkins M (1999). *Chronic Obstructive Pulmonary Disease*. Center City, MN: Hazelden Educational Materials.

O'Donoghue WJ Jr (ed.) (1995). *Long-term Oxygen Therapy*. New York: Marcel Dekker.

Useful addresses

British Lung Foundation
78 Hatton Garden
London EC1N 8LD

European Respiratory Society
1 Bd de Grancy
1006 Lausanne
Switzerland

7

Inhalation therapy

Joanna Lumb

Pharmacists have traditionally played an important role in counselling patients in the use of a wide range of drugs and appliances. The administration of drugs for the treatment of respiratory diseases is one of the prime areas where a positive input from the pharmacist can have a significant bearing on successful management of the condition. This chapter deals with the respiratory conditions in whose management pharmacists may become involved, and with the continually developing devices used for drug delivery. It should be considered as a companion to Chapter 6, which describes the use and supply of oxygen for respiratory diseases. It is not intended to provide information on the drugs used in the treatment of respiratory diseases. Information on appropriate drug treatment can be found in the current edition of the *British National Formulary*.

Most of the items used in inhalation therapy can be prescribed by the patient's doctor. Some, however, must be purchased by patients (or their families), or might be obtained on loan from the doctor's practice or a local hospital. Some patients may opt to purchase items from the local pharmacy, and it is good practice for a list of suppliers and relevant leaflets (which can be obtained from manufacturers) to be kept at the pharmacy.

Inhalation therapy is indicated for a variety of respiratory diseases. Those that will be considered here are asthma and cystic fibrosis. For a discussion of the causes and symptoms of chronic bronchitis and emphysema, see Chapter 6.

Asthma

Asthma is a chronic inflammatory disorder of the airways. It is characterised by reversible airway obstruction and increased airway responsiveness to a variety of stimuli.

Until around 10 years ago it was thought that inflammation was only present in severe disease, but it is now known that inflammatory changes are present in all asthmatic patients, whatever the severity of the disease. It appears that, in susceptible individuals, environmental factors induce a chronic mucosal inflammation characterised by eosinophil and T-cell infiltration (Figure 7.1). There is believed to be a strong genetic component to asthma.

Appreciation of the importance of inflammation has led to a change in emphasis of treatment, with increased (and earlier) use of anti-inflammatory drugs to suppress disease.

Bronchial hyperresponsiveness (an exaggerated airways response to non-specific irritants) is a consequence of the airways inflammation. It leads to clinical symptoms of wheezing and breathlessness after exposure to trigger factors (e.g. allergens, environmental irritants and viral infections).

The prevalence of asthma has steadily increased in recent years. One in 25 adults in the UK now has asthma, and one in seven children. Possible explanations for this increase include environmental pollution (e.g. exhaust fumes from cars), tobacco smoke, allergen exposure and dietary change, but evidence in support of these factors is limited.

One theory is that the increase in asthma and other atopic diseases is related to improved living conditions. This 'hygiene hypothesis' holds that reduced exposure to infections in childhood, as a consequence of improved hygiene and the widespread use of antibiotics, leads to disturbed development of the immune system and increased allergy.

Asthma can start at any age, but there are peaks of onset in child-hood and in middle age. Childhood asthma is usually associated with atopic allergy (a genetic susceptibility to produce IgE directed towards common environmental allergens); adult-onset asthma is more usually non-atopic.

Asthma used to be classified as extrinsic or intrinsic, but these terms have now largely been replaced by terms related to the asthma trigger. What was known as extrinsic asthma is now called atopic (or allergic) asthma; asthma triggered by non-allergic factors, formerly called intrinsic asthma, can be separated into categories such as exercise-induced asthma and occupational asthma.

Specific trigger factors

Inhaled allergens (antigens) are the most commonly recognised specific trigger of asthma. These allergens are proteins or glycoproteins approximately 12–25 μm in diameter which are deposited in the upper respiratory tree.

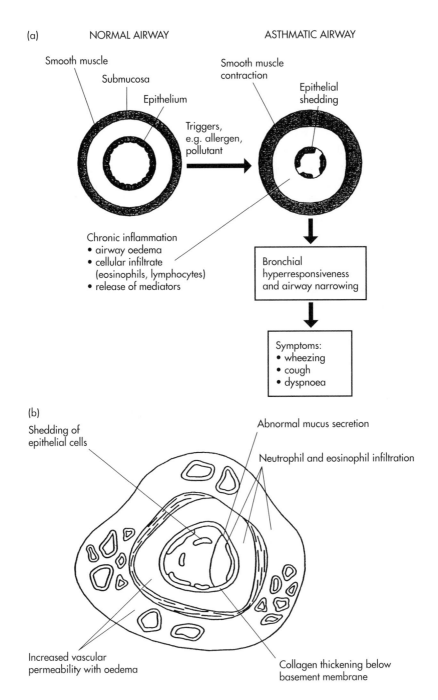

Figure 7.1 Pathology of asthma. (a) Factors that play a part in the aetiology of asthma. (b) Pathological changes in the airway in asthma. (Courtesy of Allen & Hanburys.)

The allergen stimulates the production of IgE antibodies specific for that allergen. Interaction between the allergen and IgE antibodies occurs on mast cells in the bronchial wall and leads to the release of inflammatory mediators (e.g. histamine, leukotrienes, eosinophil and neutrophil chemotactic factors, and platelet-activating factor). These mediators are associated with the early-phase asthmatic response, characterised by bronchoconstriction, which may start five to ten minutes after the antigen is inhaled; it peaks over the next 20–60 minutes and then abates. A second, often more severe, respiratory response, characterised by inflammation, oedema and mucus secretion, may occur 1–12 hours later and can last for several days. The inflammatory mediators in this late-phase asthmatic response are released from eosinophils and other cells attracted to the area.

Up to 85% of people with allergic asthma are sensitive to house dust mites. The allergen is largely found in the faecal matter of the mite. Once acquired in the home, house dust mites are virtually impossible to eradicate completely: they feed on human skin scales and live in bedding and furniture. Pet allergens, found in the pet's fur, saliva, dander, urine and faeces, are also common asthma triggers. Spores of the fungus *Aspergillus*, common in water-cooled air-conditioning systems, can also trigger asthma.

Other specific aetiological factors have been linked to the development of asthma. Allergies to chemicals in food (e.g. tartrazine) and to foods themselves (e.g. nuts, fish, dairy products and cereals) have been proposed, although food allergy is a relatively uncommon trigger for people with asthma. Occupational asthma may be associated with the production of specific IgE antibodies. Workers at risk include those who come into contact with grain, flour, tobacco, tea, silk, and synthetic and natural dyes.

Seasonal asthma may be caused by grass pollen, and to a lesser extent by tree pollen.

Non-specific trigger factors

A wide range of non-specific trigger factors for asthma has been identified, the most common being viral upper respiratory tract infection – the majority of patients with asthma find that their symptoms are triggered by viral infection. Exercise-induced asthma is characterised by bronchoconstriction during or after exercise, and the condition is most common when exercise is undertaken on cold, dry days. The type of exercise may also be important in determining the development of asthma. Of three types of exercise (cycling, swimming and running), swimming was found to be the least likely and running the most likely to provoke a response. Patients with exercise-induced asthma are advised to take a dose of 'reliever' medication before starting exercise.

Sudden changes in temperature, cold air, windy weather, humidity, dampness and poor air quality on dry still days are all common triggers for people with asthma. Thunderstorms have been reported to trigger symptoms. There is little evidence that air pollution causes asthma but it does make symptoms worse for many patients. Although dry air may be a factor in the development of asthma, the uncontrolled use of humidifiers can be counterproductive. Humidifiers can readily become contaminated with microorganisms whose distribution in the atmosphere may provoke bronchoconstriction.

Drug-induced asthma can be predicted on a pharmacological basis. Non-cardioselective β-adrenoceptor blocking drugs used in the treatment of cardiovascular disease and glaucoma can lead to asthmatic attacks through their action on the β_2 bronchial receptors. Iodinated contrast media and other drugs (e.g. non-steroidal anti-inflammatories) can provoke a similar response. Between 4 and 20% of patients with asthma are reported to be sensitive to aspirin. Paradoxical bronchoconstriction has been reported with a number of inhaled medicines used for treating asthma. This is thought to result from non-specific irritation of the bronchial mucosa. The problem has occurred with both metered-dose inhalers and nebuliser solutions.

Asthmatic symptoms may become worse in women immediately before or at the onset of menstruation. Evidence for a hormonal component is strengthened by an unpredictable general improvement or worsening of symptoms during pregnancy.

Clinical presentation

Asthma is associated with episodes of wheezing, breathlessness, chest tightness and coughing, particularly at night and in the early morning. Breathlessness is typically described by patients as an inability to get air out of their lungs. Cough is often accompanied by excess production of sputum, which is purulent even in the absence of upper respiratory tract infection, and can cause distress, particularly at night.

A diurnal pattern of symptom occurrence has been identified. Measurement of peak expiratory flow rate (see Lung function tests, below) indicates that many asthmatic patients have the greatest degree of airways obstruction between 0200 and 0400 h. This has been associated with high circulating levels of histamine and low levels of adrenaline, and the symptoms may be severe enough to wake the patient.

In children there may be a history of infantile eczema or rhinitis, and parents may describe a cold which has 'gone on to the chest'. Exercise performance may be below that of other children of the same age and there may be growth impairment, especially in boys. In non-smoking adults, late-onset asthma may be characterised by wheeze early in the morning. Cough and sputum may be present, and there may be a history of childhood allergy or hay fever.

In both adults and children increased and potentially life-threatening symptoms may be characterised by anxiety, distress, disturbed sleep and cyanosis. Severe respiratory embarrassment may be accompanied by tachypnoea, tachycardia and pulsus paradoxus (an exaggerated variation in the normal cyclical fluctuations in systolic blood pressure which occurs during the respiratory cycle). During a severe attack patients may be unable to talk.

Death is rare, but when it does occur it usually does so at night and is unexpected. Patients at higher risk of a severe attack of acute asthma include those who have had a previous episode within the past few months and those whose compliance with dosage schedules has lapsed. Despite the availability of effective treatment, the mortality rate from asthma has not fallen significantly. Poor compliance, overreliance on bronchodilator therapy, underuse of anti-inflammatory therapy and lack of peak flow monitoring are among factors that have been suggested to be associated with 'avoidable' deaths. The importance of input from the pharmacist is emphasised by suggestions that many patients do not understand their complex drug regimens (e.g. they do not appreciate the reasons for regular prophylactic treatment) and fail to use their inhalation products correctly.

Cystic fibrosis

Cystic fibrosis is the most common life-threatening genetically inherited disorder in white populations; it rarely occurs in Asians or Africans. The disease is inherited in a mendelian recessive manner, requiring both parents to be carriers of the defective gene. It is equally common in males and females. If both parents are asymptomatic carriers of the gene, a child has a one in four chance of inheriting cystic fibrosis. Children from two carrier-state parents also have a 50% chance of becoming carriers, and of subsequently passing the gene to their own offspring (Figure 7.2).

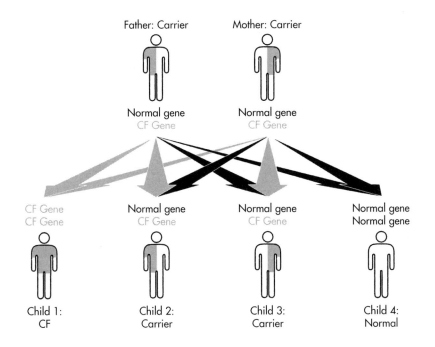

Figure 7.2 Inheritance of cystic fibrosis: a baby can be born with CF only if both parents are carriers of the CF gene. (Courtesy of the Cystic Fibrosis Trust.)

It has been estimated that about 1 in 25 people in the UK are carriers of the gene and that about 1 partnership in 500 consists of two carriers. One in every 2500 babies in the UK is born with cystic fibrosis.

The cystic fibrosis gene is located on chromosome 7. It makes a protein called cystic fibrosis transmembrane conductance regulator (CFTR), which controls chloride ion transport across cell surfaces. Some 800 different mutations of the cystic fibrosis gene have been described, but 80% of cases in the UK are associated with one particular mutation, δ F508.

The identification of the cystic fibrosis gene offers the prospect of curing the disease by corrrecting the basic gene defect. In theory, the faulty gene could be replaced with a healthy copy. Early trials have provided proof of principle that gene therapy may work, but results so far have been too short-lived to be of clinical benefit.

Screening and diagnosis

Carrier testing

Population screening of adults for carrier status is currently not recommended. However, testing may be offered to prospective parents if a relative has cystic fibrosis or is a known carrier. Screening usually involves a mouthwash test.

Antenatal diagnosis

Antenatal screening may be undertaken in pregnancies in which there is a high risk of the birth of a child with cystic fibrosis. Testing generally involves chorionic villus sampling in around the tenth week of pregnancy for DNA analysis. The procedure carries a small but definite risk of miscarriage.

Neonatal screening

Early detection and treatment of cystic fibrosis by routine screening for the disease in newborn infants (using a heel-prick blood test) can help to prevent lung damage and avoid malnutrition. Screening is currently not available in many parts of the UK, but the government has announced plans to extend the screening programme.

Diagnosis

Most people with cystic fibrosis are diagnosed by two years of age. The classic diagnostic test for cystic fibrosis involves the detection of abnormally high levels of sodium and chloride in a sweat sample collected following pilocarpine iontophoresis of a small area of skin. Values of sodium or chloride in excess of 60 mmol/L are diagnostic of cystic fibrosis. The presence of excess salt in sweat is caused by a malfunction in the ability to absorb salt as the sweat passes up towards the surface of the skin.

Clinical presentation

Cystic fibrosis is a multisystem disease, as CFTR is widespread though the body, but the two major systems affected are the lungs and the gastrointestinal tract.

About one in six patients with cystic fibrosis is identified by the presence of meconium ileus in the neonate. This is characterised by blockage of the small intestine, which might have to be relieved surgically. However, most children with the disease are identified by recurrent respiratory tract infections or by signs of pancreatic enzyme deficiency (steatorrhoea and a failure to thrive).

Impaired ion transport makes the airway secretions very viscous and predisposes the patient to chronic bacterial infection and lung damage. Respiratory problems may begin soon after birth as a slight cough. As the child gets older, recurrent lower respiratory tract infections can lead to bronchiectasis. The predominant pathogens in childhood are *Staphylococcus aureus* and, less frequently, *Haemophilus influenzae*; chronic colonisation with *Pseudomonas aeruginosa* is common by the late teens. Wheeze and breathlessness can also cause problems.

Some degree of pancreatic insufficiency occurs in over 90% of patients. The pancreatic duct becomes blocked by a viscid mucus, and the back-pressure on the pancreas results in the destruction of gland tissue. Pancreatic insufficiency leads to malabsorption, with steatorrhoea and the passage of foul-smelling, greasy stools. The unpleasant smell is produced by the presence of partially digested protein. CF-related diabetes mellitus occurs in up to 25% of patients.

The ileum can become partially blocked by a solid or semisolid mass, which may cause constipation, abdominal pain and distension. The blockage can be precipitated by dehydration as a consequence of respiratory tract infection, or by poor compliance with the administration of pancreatic enzyme supplements.

Reproductive function is severely affected. The majority of men are infertile, owing to abnormality of the vas deferens. Many women with cystic fibrosis can become pregnant despite the presence of thickened cervical mucus. However, lung function can deteriorate rapidly during pregnancy.

Management

The management of cystic fibrosis involves drug therapy, nutrition and physiotherapy.

Nutritional management is essential because of the absence of pancreatic enzymes and the resultant malabsorption. Pancreatic insufficiency is treated with oral pancreatic enzyme supplements containing amylase, lipase and protease. Supplements of fat-soluble vitamins are also usually required.

Even in the presence of pancreatic enzyme supplements food may be inadequately digested and absorbed, and increased intake may be needed to compensate. It is imperative that a good nutritional status is maintained to minimise the risks of the development of respiratory tract infections. The precise extra quantity of food necessary for growth (in children) and maintenance of health varies considerably, and patients will be advised by a dietitian. As fat provides an excellent source of energy, low-fat diets are not recommended. The range of dietary products that can be given to treat malabsorption is described in Chapter 8.

In cystic fibrosis, antibiotics are given orally, intravenously and by nebuliser. Prophylactic long-term nebulised antibiotics are given to patients with chronic *Pseudomonas* colonisation, with courses of intravenous antibiotics for acute exacerbations. Home intravenous antibiotic treatment is often possible nowadays. Some patients who need regular intravenous antibiotics may be fitted with an implantable venous access device, which is positioned on the chest wall or upper arm and can be left in place for several years. Community pharmacists should be aware of the syringe drivers and portable infusion devices used for home intravenous treatment, but the patient's care will be monitored by the hospital cystic fibrosis team.

Physiotherapy is an integral part of patient management and should be carried out twice daily. The techniques are taught to parents of babies and young children and may be used even in the absence of symptoms of respiratory obstruction. Older children and adults are taught procedures which they can perform for themselves.

Lung function tests

Lung function tests are invaluable in the diagnosis of obstructive lung disease, in assessing the severity of a patient's condition and in monitoring the effectiveness of a prescribed regimen.

Spirometric testing can be carried out in hospital and general practice. These tests allow the calculation of forced vital capacity (FVC, the volume of air that can be forcefully exhaled), forced expiratory volume in one second (FEV_1), and the ratio of FEV_1 to FVC, which is expressed as a percentage and has a normal value of about 75%. (Normal values vary according to race, height, age and sex.) In obstructive airways disease FEV_1 is reduced more than FVC, and so the FEV_1/FVC ratio is reduced. In restrictive lung disease both FVC and FEV_1 are reduced and the ratio is normal or elevated. Spirometry can also be used to measure the reversibility of airways obstruction, by taking measurements before and after use of a bronchodilator.

In the home, much cheaper alternatives are available that permit regular testing of respiratory function. The simplest and cheapest measurement that can be taken is the peak expiratory flow rate (PEFR), a reading of the maximum flow of air when the patient is breathing out as hard as possible. In practice, the maximum velocity of air flow is achieved early in expiration. The standard device used for measuring PEFR is the peak flow meter. The patient blows into the mouthpiece, forcing an indicator tab along a graduated slot; the tab remains at the maximum level for the reading to be noted by the patient or parent (Figure 7.3).

Readings should be taken at the same time each day. It is recommended that the patient practise blowing into the device by taking a couple of deep breaths without emptying the lungs. Three successive 'full-blow' attempts can then be made and the highest reading of the three recorded on a chart. The record chart serves two purposes. It enables the patient's doctor to monitor variations in the degree of bronchoconstriction (e.g. produced early in the morning or related to work) and it helps patients to 'manage' their own condition by responding to changes in lung function.

Peak flow monitoring is not necessary for all patients. However, it may be recommended as part of the self-management plan for adults and older children who are poor perceivers of symptoms (and hence slow to detect deterioration in their asthma), for those with severe or 'brittle' asthma, or to monitor the effects of changes in treatment. Patients must be advised on action to take if their peak flow falls below a certain level.

Peak flow meters are prescribable on FP10. The devices are available in standard and low range. The standard-range meters are suitable for the majority of adults and children, whereas the lower-range meters are designed for adults and children with severely reduced peak flow. Most adults and children over six years of age can use a peak flow meter.

Principles of inhalation therapy

It is advantageous to deliver a drug for the treatment of respiratory disease direct to the required site of action. A smaller dose can be given than by the oral route of administration, and as a result the incidence of side-effects can be reduced. Inhalation therapy also permits more rapid delivery to the lungs than systemic routes of administration.

In the past 10–15 years the types of drugs used to treat asthma have changed relatively little, but there have been significant developments in

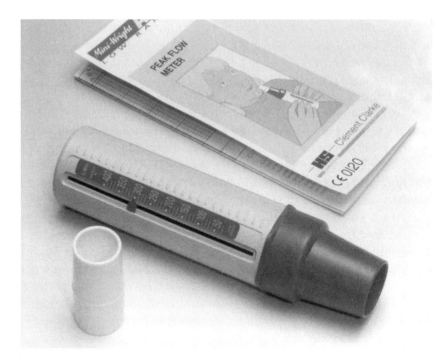

SECTION 2.
Record your peak flow by
using your peak flow meter in
the morning and evening.
Mark a cross on the graph
against the score for the best
of three blows.

Figure 7.3 Peak flow meter (courtesy of Clement Clarke) and sample record chart
(courtesy of Allen & Hanburys).

the devices available for their delivery to the lungs. Pharmacists can help
to ensure that the most appropriate device is chosen and that patients
have accurate information on their use.

In order to obtain therapeutic levels of inhaled drugs, the particle size of the administered agent must be carefully controlled. The lungs act to minimise the inward penetration of particles, and normal defence mechanisms are equally effective in excluding particles from inhaled dosage forms. The critical factors for drug inhalation therapy are the shape, size and density of inhaled particles. These factors are characterised by the mass median aerodynamic diameter (MMAD). Particles with an MMAD in excess of 10 µm do not penetrate further than the upper respiratory tract. Particles are extracted from the airstream through impaction and are removed to the gastrointestinal tract by swallowing. Particles of 5–10 µm diameter pass through the larynx, but the turbulence experienced immediately below it results in further particle impaction. The mucus and beating cilia in this region carry impacted particles towards the pharynx, where they are swallowed.

Smaller particles of 1–5 µm diameter may pass through the trachea and enter and penetrate deep within the bronchi. They are large enough to be deposited by gravity on the walls of the respiratory tree, but not so small that they are immediately removed on exhalation. Deposited particles of soluble drug subsequently dissolve and may enter the cells of the bronchi and alveoli to exert their therapeutic effect.

It has been estimated that only about 5–20% of the inhaled dose reaches the required site of action deep within the lungs. The proportion can be further reduced by poor inhalation technique, and a variety of devices have been developed in attempts to improve the delivery of drugs to the lungs.

Metered-dose inhalers

Metered-dose inhalers (MDIs) containing drugs for the prevention and treatment of respiratory disease have been available since the early 1960s and are still the most commonly prescribed inhaler device for treatment of asthma. They are small and unobtrusive and can easily be carried by the patient, to be available as required. They are multidose devices containing about 200 doses in each unit. The drug is contained within a pressurised sealed aluminium canister and may be present as a solution or suspension in about 10 mL of propellant. A wetting agent may also be present to prevent the agglomeration of particles of suspended drug. The canister is mounted upside-down in a plastic actuator, and a small metering chamber is located at the bottom of the canister. When the canister is not in use, this metering chamber is open to the rest of the canister. When the inverted canister is pressed on from above, the metering chamber becomes sealed from the rest of the canister but open to the atmosphere. As a result, about 10–50 µL of the pressurised material is released through a narrow opening into the air. Passage through the narrow orifice helps to disrupt the suspension/solution into a stream of rapidly moving droplets. The drug is surrounded by droplets of propellant, which evaporate as the drug particles pass through the air. As a significant amount of the propellant evaporates, the average particle size of the spray falls dramatically, producing particles of the size range required to enter the lower respiratory tree.

The amount of drug released on actuation varies with each drug administered by this route. It must also be borne in mind, however, that only 5–20% of each actuation dose reaches the site of action of the drug (see above), and that a large proportion of each dose is lost to the atmosphere.

Until the late 1990s MDIs contained chlorofluorocarbon (CFC) propellants. However, because of the recognition that CFCs destroy stratospheric ozone, an international agreement was reached to stop their use (the Montreal Protocol 1987), and new hydrofluoroalkane (HFA) propellants have been developed for use in asthma inhalers. These are much less damaging than CFCs to the earth's ozone layer.

The first CFC-free inhaler was introduced in 1995. Others are being phased in, and eventually all MDIs will be CFC free. Patients need to be reassured that the change is being made for environmental reasons rather than for clinical or safety reasons. The new inhalers are designed to be used in the same way as CFC-containing MDIs. However, differences in the physicochemical properties of the propellants mean that patients swapping to the new inhalers may notice that they feel or taste different from their CFC inhaler.

The effective administration of drugs by MDIs is strongly dependent on inhaler technique. For the drug to be delivered to the lower respiratory tree, it is essential that the patient synchronises actuation of the inhaler with inhalation. Many studies have shown that tuition in the use of MDIs can significantly improve the development of correct technique. Equally, reinforcing the instruction when repeat prescriptions are presented has been shown to ensure continued correct technique. It is essential that, whenever practicable, the pharmacist checks that the patient is fully aware of the appropriate technique. Pharmacists should be alert to increased frequency or quantities of repeat prescriptions from patients with MDIs, as these may indicate a deterioration in the condition (when the patient should be referred for consultation with the doctor) or poor technique requiring more frequent use of the drug to alleviate symptoms (when reinforcement training in technique may be appropriate). Some companies supply placebo training devices with which the pharmacist can demonstrate correct procedures. These could be used on initial presentation of a prescription, and at regular intervals thereafter.

One disadvantage of MDIs is that there is no facility to show how many doses are left in the device.

Inhaler technique

The following steps are recommended by the National Asthma and Respiratory Training Centre for satisfactory delivery of a drug from a standard MDI:

1. Remove the cap.
2. Shake the inhaler.
3. Breathe out gently.
4. Put the mouthpiece in the mouth and, at the start of inspiration, which should be slow and deep, press the canister down and continue to inhale deeply.
5. Hold the breath for 10 seconds, or as long as possible, then breathe out slowly.
6. Wait for a few seconds before repeating steps 2–5.
7. Replace cap.

A significant proportion of patients, particularly children and the elderly, have problems mastering the coordination required between actuation and inspiration. Patients may actuate the device during expiration, or before the start or after the completion of inspiration. They may breathe in through the nose rather than the mouth. Some patients may be uncertain whether the drug has been released and may actuate the device more than once during a single inspiration. Another problem is that some patients may gag or stop inhaling when the propellant hits the back of the throat (the 'cold freon' effect). This effect should be reduced with CFC-free inhalers, as the propellant leaves the inhaler more slowly and is warmer.

Breath-actuated pressurised MDIs

These devices (e.g. Autohaler, Easi-Breathe) are designed for patients who have problems coordinating actuation and inhalation with a standard MDI. The devices are primed before each actuation, either by opening the cap (Easi-Breathe) or by moving a lever (Autohaler). A single dose is then released when the patient inhales (Figure 7.4).

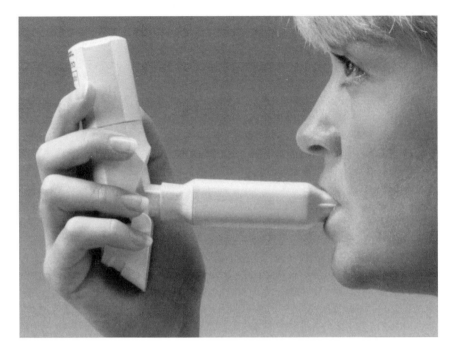

Figure 7.4 Easi-Breathe breath-actuated inhaler with extension tube. (Courtesy of IVAX Pharmaceuticals UK.)

Spacer devices

Two types of spacer device are available to help patients using MDIs: extension devices and valved holding chambers. They reduce the oropharyngeal deposition of drug by slowing the aerosol and allowing the propellants to evaporate, thereby reducing the size of the aerosol droplets and trapping large particles in the spacer.

Extension devices are supplied with some pressurised MDIs. These devices do not have a valve, and coordination of actuation and inspiration is still required for optimal drug delivery.

Valved holding chambers, generally referred to as spacers, have a one-way valve and a reservoir into which the drug is released from the aerosol canister (Figures 7.5 and 7.6). The patient can inhale the drug from the spacer in their own time, without the need to coordinate actuation and inspiration. The use of valved holding chambers is recommended for all patients using high-dose steroids. The possibility of the propellant producing the 'cold freon' effect (see above) is eliminated.

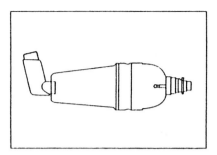

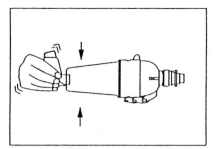

1a. Remove the mouthpiece from the adapter.

1b. Place the adapter into the oval opening of the inhalation chamber.

2. Shake the aerosol canister so that the contents of the canister are mixed well. Next push the aerosol canister into Nebuhaler via the adaptor, as shown in the diagram.

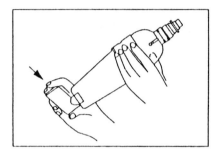

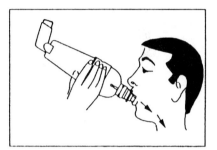

3. Hold Nebuhaler pointing slightly downwards, as shown in the picture. Press the canister to release one puff into the inhalation chamber.

4. Place the mouthpiece between your teeth, close your lips and breathe in slowly and deeply through your mouth. This is to make sure that the medicine has been emptied from Nebuhaler.

If more than one puff has been prescribed, repeat steps 3–4.
If you use Pulmicort: rinse your mouth out with water after each dosing occasion.

Figure 7.5 Nebuhaler usage instructions. (Courtesy of AstraZeneca UK.)

Spacers are becoming increasingly popular for the delivery of inhaled drugs in the treatment of asthma. Face masks allow them to be used by infants and children too young to use a mouthpiece. Drug delivery via a mouthpiece is more efficient, however, and should be used in preference to a face mask as early as possible.

The use of an MDI with a spacer has been shown to be as effective as nebulisers in the treatment of acute asthma.

Spacers vary in size from 135 mL to 750 mL. Not all spacers are prescribable on FP10.

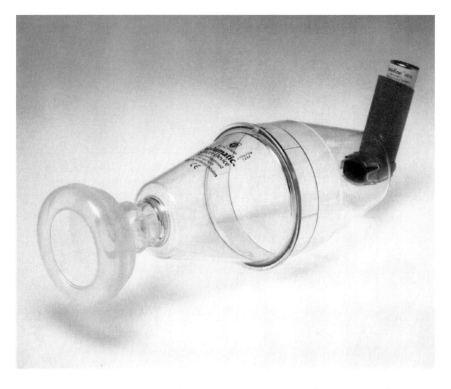

Figure 7.6 Volumatic spacer device with mask attached. (Courtesy of Allen & Hanburys.)

Advice for using holding chamber spacers

The following advice should be adhered to when using chamber spacers:

- If the patient needs more than one dose of drug, repeated single actuations of the MDI into the spacer should be made, each followed by inhalation. Multiple actuations into the spacer before inhalation may reduce the proportion of dose inhaled.
- It is important to keep delay to a minimum between actuation and inhalation. A delay of only five seconds has been shown to reduce the amount of drug available for inhalation.
- Static electricity can accumulate on plastic and polycarbonate spacers, attracting drug particles and reducing the amount of drug delivered. Regular washing of the spacer can reduce this. Spacers should be washed in a household detergent and allowed to air dry without rinsing. If there are concerns about the possibility of

contact dermatitis using this method, the mouthpiece or face mask should be rinsed in water and dried.

Manufacturers provide specific instructions about washing their spacers.

Not all spacers are compatible with all pressurised MDIs. The choice of spacer for the chosen MDI should be guided by the information in the Summary of Product Characteristics. The UK Department of Health says that it should not be assumed that a combination of spacer device and CFC-free MDI will be equivalent to the same combination using the CFC product, because of possible differences in electrostatic interactions between the new formulation and the spacer.

Breath-operated powder inhalers

Dry powder inhalers do not use a propellant but rely on the patient's inspiratory flow to disperse the drug into small particles and deliver it to the lungs. Some devices require loading with drug before each use, or every few doses, which can require dexterity. The more recently introduced disposable multidose devices do not require loading.

As with MDIs, dry powder devices can be associated with oropharyngeal deposition of drug.

Unit-dose powder inhalers

These devices (Spinhaler and Rotahaler) require loading before each dose. A micronised powder, with or without an inert powdered diluent, is contained within a hard gelatin capsule. The capsule is placed within a device that pierces the capsule or separates it into two halves to release the powder.

Multidose powder inhalers

Multidose devices are now much more commonly used than the unit-dose inhalers.

With some inhalers (e.g. Diskhaler and Aerohaler), premeasured doses are loaded by the patient into reusable devices. Diskhalers are used with micronised powdered drug (plus lactose carrier) contained in hermetically sealed foil blisters. The blisters (four or eight) are arranged on a circular aluminium foil disc which is inserted into a piercing and delivery device (the Diskhaler) (Figure 7.7). The drug is released from a single compartment by the patient before each dose is administered. This is

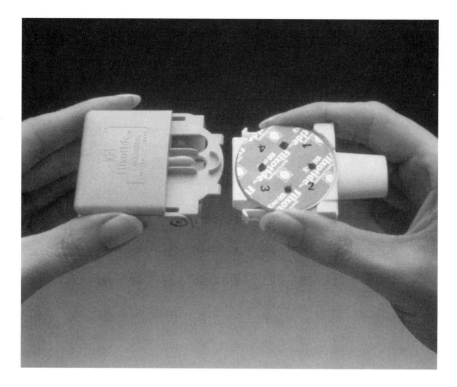

Figure 7.7 Diskhaler dry powder inhaler. (Courtesy of Allen & Hanburys.)

achieved by raising an integral flap which pierces the upper and lower surfaces of the blister with a needle. The rotating disc incorporates an indicator which advises the patient of the number of remaining doses.

With the Aerohaler device the drug (mixed with glucose) is supplied in hard gelatin capsules, up to six of which can be loaded at a time. Patients should only load the number of capsules they need for that day, as once capsules are removed from the foil blister pack they must be used within one day. Pushing a trigger button on the side of the device pierces a capsule so the drug is ready for inhalation (Figure 7.8). A marker shows how many doses are still available in the device.

The concept of multidose powder inhalers was extended with the introduction of disposable multidose metered-dose powder inhalers (Turbohaler, Accuhaler and Clickhaler), which do not need loading by the patient. They all indicate with a red warning when just a few doses are left.

In the Turbohaler, the drug powder is stored in a gravity-fed powder reservoir holding up to 200 doses. The device requires no manual

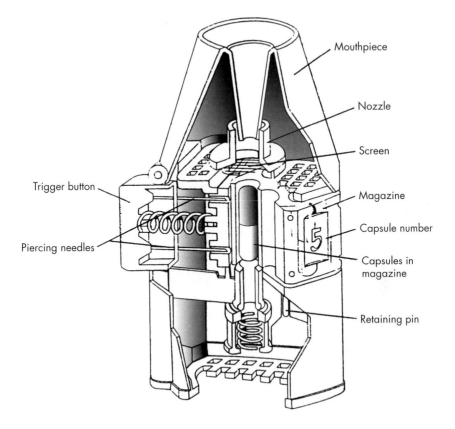

Mouthpiece

Nozzle

Screen

Trigger button

Magazine

Capsule number

Piercing needles

Capsules in magazine

Retaining pin

Figure 7.8 Internal diagram of the Aerohaler dry powder device. (Courtesy of Boehringer Ingelheim.)

operation other than the removal of the outer protective cover and a simple twist of the base back and forth before use. This twisting fills a number of conical holes in a rotating disc with the drug. Scrapers then remove surplus drug as the disc passes beneath them, to ensure accurate dosage. As the patient inhales, the powder is deaggregated by turbulence and a mouthpiece insert. A dessicant is stored in the base of the Turbohaler.

The Clickhaler, which looks rather like an MDI, contains 200 doses. Micronised drug (plus lactose) is contained in a hopper and a metered dose is delivered from the bulk powder on actuation. The device uses dimples in a frustoconical metering cone to transfer fixed amounts of bulk powder from a reservoir into the airstream. A Venturi effect lifts and deaggregates the powder, which is then swept down a boot-shaped mouthpiece. Pushing a button actuates the metering cone.

The Accuhaler is a moulded plastic device containing a foil strip with 60 regularly placed blisters containing drug (plus lactose). The individual blisters are opened as the device is manipulated. Pushing a lever primes the device. When the patient inhales, air passages draw air in through the body top, into the manifold and through the opened blister, dispersing the contents and delivering the dose via the mouthpiece to the patient. Two holes in the mouthpiece draw in more air, creating further turbulence as the dose leaves the mouthpiece (Figure 7.9).

Choosing an inhaler

The best choice of inhaler is one that the patient will use on a regular basis and in an effective manner. For adults, the selection of an appropriate

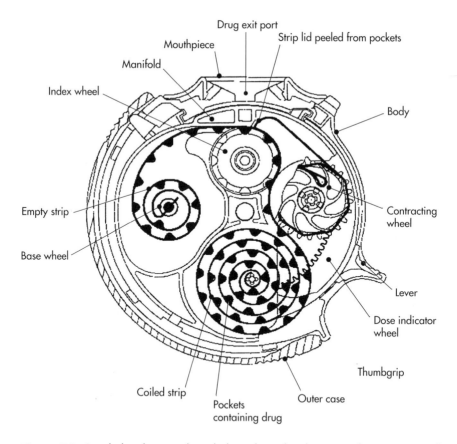

Figure 7.9 Accuhaler dry powder inhaler – how the device works. (Courtesy of Allen & Hanburys.)

device depends largely on individual preference and the ease with which the device can be operated. MDIs are often the first choice for adults, with a spacer recommended for high-dose steroids and for any patient who has difficulty with coordination.

Children form a large group of patients to whom inhalation therapy is given. The effectiveness of therapy depends on the ease with which they can operate inhalation devices. It has been suggested that pressurised MDIs cannot generally be used efficiently without a spacer by children under about 12 years of age. Breath-actuated MDIs and dry powder devices might be used at an earlier age.

Specific guidance on inhaler choice for treating chronic stable asthma in children under five years of age was issued by the National Institute for Clinical Excellence (NICE) in 2000. NICE recommendations are as follows:

- Use of a pressurised MDI and spacer system, with a face mask where necessary (allowing the child to inhale the drug over several breaths).
- If this is not clinically effective, and depending on the child's condition, nebulised therapy may be considered.
- For children aged three to five years, a dry powder inhaler might also be considered.

A device called In-check Dial is marketed to help inhaler selection. This is a handheld inspiratory flow measurement device which can simulate the internal resistance of different dry powder devices and breath-actuated MDIs and is used to check which devices the patient will most easily be able to use.

Patient information and inhaler aids

Manufacturers provide detailed leaflets to explain the use of their inhalers to patients, and these leaflets often also incorporate explanatory diagrams. Pharmacists must be aware of the content of these leaflets before discussing them with patients. It is also vital that time is spent with the patient when a prescription is first presented, to reinforce any advice given by the doctor or nurse. The use of placebo devices may help patients to understand verbal and written instructions. As many powder inhalers are used by young children unable to provide the coordination necessary for an MDI, it is also important for parents or carers to be fully competent in the techniques.

The National Asthma and Respiratory Training Centre has produced a series of laminated cards illustrating use of different inhaler devices (Figure 7.10). These are available for purchase.

Patients should be advised to follow the manufacturers' instructions on cleaning their inhalers.

Some patients using MDIs may have difficulty holding the device and simultaneously depressing the base of the canister. An attachment (the Haleraid) is available to alleviate this problem for patients with arthritis or others with poor manual dexterity. The device is placed around the plastic actuator case and squeezed to deliver the dose. It is available in two sizes to fit different sized MDIs. The Turboaid is a device which can be attached to the Turbohaler to improve grip. Neither of these aids is available on NHS prescription.

HOW TO USE A METERED DOSE INHALER

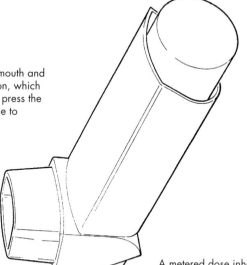

1. Remove the cap.

2. Shake the inhaler.

3. Breathe out gently.

4. Put the mouthpiece in the mouth and at the start of the inspiration, which should be slow and deep, press the canister down and continue to inhale deeply.

5. Hold the breath for 10 seconds, or as long as possible, then breathe out slowly.

6. Wait for a few seconds before repeating steps 2–5.

7. Replace cap.

A metered dose inhaler

ALWAYS DEMONSTRATE TO THE PATIENT HOW TO USE THE METERED DOSE INHALER

© NATIONAL ASTHMA & RESPIRATORY TRAINING CENTRE, WARWICK

Figure 7.10 Inhaler technique: instruction cards produced by the National Asthma and Respiratory Training Centre.

EMERGENCY TREATMENT VIA SPACER DEVICE

1. Put 2 parts of spacer together.

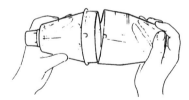

2. Remove cap of inhaler.

3. Shake inhaler.

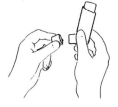

4. Insert inhaler into flat end of device.

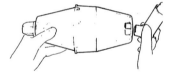

5. Place mouthpiece in patient's mouth and press inhaler canister once to release a dose of the reliever medication.

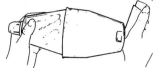

6. Tell the patient to breathe in and out. Repeat step 5, with device in mouth, allowing 4–5 breaths between actuations.

7. Shake the inhaler between every actuation. 10–20 puffs, one at a time, can be used depending on age.

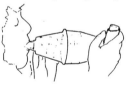

8. Remove the device from mouth.

**SEEK HELP IF CONDITION IS NOT RELIEVED WITHIN 5 MINUTES
WHILE HELP IS BEING SOUGHT REPEAT STAGES 5–7**

© NATIONAL ASTHMA & RESPIRATORY TRAINING CENTRE, WARWICK

Figure 7.10 Inhaler technique: instruction cards produced by the National Asthma and Respiratory Training Centre.

Nebulisers

A nebuliser is a device which converts a drug solution into an aerosol that can be inhaled into the lungs. The aim is to deliver a therapeutic dose in the form of respirable particles (1–5 µm) within a fairly short period of time.

The use of nebulisers in asthma has declined in recent years, largely because of research (mentioned earlier) showing that acute attacks of

HOW TO USE THE TURBOHALER

Turbohaler

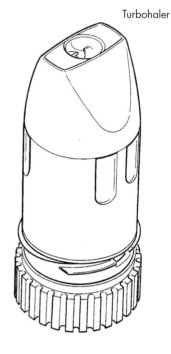

1. Unscrew and lift off white cover.

2. Hold Turbohaler upright and twist the grip then twist it back again as far as it will go. You should hear a click.

3. Breathe out gently, put the mouthpiece between the lips and teeth and breathe in as deeply as possible. Even when a full dose is taken there may be no taste (do not breathe out into Turbohaler).

4. Remove the Turbohaler from the mouth and hold breath for about 10 seconds.

5. For a second dose repeat steps 2–4.

6. Replace white cover.

7. A red line appears in the window on the side of the Turbohaler when there are 20 doses left. When the whole window is red the inhaler is empty.

ALWAYS DEMONSTRATE TO THE PATIENT HOW TO USE THE TURBOHALER

© NATIONAL ASTHMA & RESPIRATORY TRAINING CENTRE, WARWICK

Figure 7.10 Inhaler technique: instruction cards produced by the National Asthma and Respiratory Training Centre.

asthma in both adults and children can be treated as effectively with multiple doses of bronchodilator given by MDI and spacer as with a nebuliser. Nebulisers can, however, be useful when large doses of drug are needed, or when patients are too ill or otherwise unable to use a hand-held inhaler.

The most common indication for nebulisers is for bronchodilatation in the emergency treatment of asthma and exacerbations of chronic obstructive pulmonary disease. Nebulisation is less frequently used for prophylactic drug treatment (e.g. using steroids and sodium cromoglycate). In cystic fibrosis, nebulised treatment can include antibiotics, saline (perhaps with bronchodilators) before physiotherapy to help clear secretions, and dornase alfa to reduce sputum viscosity.

HOW TO USE THE ACCUHALER

1. Open the Accuhaler by holding the outer casing in one hand while pushing the thumbgrip away until a click is heard.

2. Hold the Accuhaler with the mouthpiece towards you, slide the lever away until it clicks. This makes the dose available for inhalation and moves the dose counter on.

3. Holding the Accuhaler level, breathe out gently away from the device, put mouthpiece in mouth and take a breath in steadily and deeply.

4. Remove the Accuhaler from mouth and hold breath for about 10 seconds.

5. To close, slide the thumbgrip back towards you as far as it will go until it clicks.

6. For a second dose, repeat steps 1–5.

7. The dose counter counts down from 60 to 0. The last 5 numbers are red

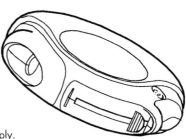

Accuhaler

ALWAYS DEMONSTRATE TO THE PATIENT HOW TO USE THE ACCUHALER

© NATIONAL ASTHMA & RESPIRATORY TRAINING CENTRE, WARWICK

Figure 7.10 Inhaler technique: instruction cards produced by the National Asthma and Respiratory Training Centre.

The two major types of nebulising device are the ultrasonic nebuliser and the jet nebuliser, the latter being more commonly used. In the UK, nebulisers for domiciliary use are not available at NHS expense. Although drugs administered with a nebuliser must be obtained on a doctor's prescription, concern has been expressed at the potential misuse of these devices in the home. Asthmatic patients, in particular, may rely too much on their use and delay seeking medical help (e.g. during an acute attack).

If pharmacists are involved in the supply of solutions to be used in a nebuliser, they should be aware of the procedures for the effective use of these devices. They must also be capable of giving advice if patients are experiencing difficulties in the control of the condition. This responsibility should be particularly borne in mind if the pharmacist is the supplier of the nebuliser apparatus.

Ultrasonic nebulisers

Ultrasonic nebulisers work on the principle of a high-frequency vibration which separates liquid into small droplets. The vibration is generated by the passage of an electric current through a ceramic disc (piezoelectric transducer). The disc varies in thickness in response to the alternating current, and this establishes a wave pattern through the liquid lying above it. If a high-frequency electrical source is used (e.g. 1–2 mHz), the liquid will be disrupted to produce droplets of about 5 μm diameter.

Compared with jet nebulisers, ultrasonic nebulisers are virtually silent when running and do not require an external source of compressed gas. A high volume of the drug is quickly delivered and there is considerably less wastage than with traditional jet nebulisers. However, ultrasonic nebulisers are generally more expensive and less robust than jet nebulisers and they are not used for regular domiciliary therapy.

Jet nebulisers

Jet nebulisers consist of a nebulising chamber in which an aerosol is generated by a flow of gas from an electrical compressor or from a compressed gas supply (air or oxygen). The nebuliser produces an aerosol through a Venturi effect generated by a Bernoulli nozzle. The driving gas enters the chamber through a tube whose opening is restricted. The restriction creates a jet stream of high velocity and this is directed across the end of a fine capillary tube, the other end of which is immersed in a solution of the drug to be nebulised. The high velocity of the gas stream creates an area of negative pressure within the tube. This effect, coupled to the presence of normal atmospheric pressure bearing down on the liquid reservoir, forces fluid up the capillary tube. At the end of the tube the liquid is caught in the stream of gas and broken into droplets of varying size, producing a fine spray.

An appropriate distribution of particle sizes for inhalation into the lower respiratory tree is produced by the action of an obstacle: a baffle. Large droplets are selectively removed by the change in direction of flow produced by the baffle and these coalesce and run back down into the liquid reservoir. The shape of the baffle determines the particle size distribution and density of the spray that enters the patient's lungs. Larger particles which bypass removal by the baffle may be extracted by impact with other internal surfaces of the nebuliser. This process of condensation may also have important consequences for determining the duration of 'continuous' nebulisation that may be achieved. Most nebulisers use only small volumes of solution (e.g. 4 mL) and, if a large proportion of the droplets produced coalesces, there may be a period when no spray is passed to the lungs ('intermittent' nebulisation). This may be seen as a fizzing in the nebuliser solution. Tapping the sides of the nebuliser may encourage the coalesced drops to run back into the liquid reservoir. The selection of a suitably powerful driving source for the gas stream is critical to ensure continuous nebulisation.

For home use, an air compressor is used to provide the driving gas. Domiciliary oxygen cylinders do not provide an adequate flow rate. Compressors may be electric or battery operated. A flow rate of between 6 and 8 L/min is normally needed to drive the nebuliser. Domiciliary compressors usually provide a continuous air flow. It is imperative to select a compressor that is appropriate for driving a particular nebuliser. The manufacturer's literature should be consulted for this information.

A foot-operated pump may be suitable (e.g. when the patient is on holiday at a site without a power supply). Some foot pumps can deliver 2 mL of solution in three minutes, but a more common delivery period is six to eight minutes. However, the physical effort needed to drive the nebuliser over a minimum period of five minutes is considerable, and may be impossible for a person lacking good respiratory drive.

Conventional jet nebulisers are easy to use but inefficient in drug delivery, only around 10% of prescribed drug reaching the lungs. There is constant output of aerosol from the nebuliser during both inspiration and expiration. This means that a large amount of drug is wasted as it is produced during expiration.

Several new nebulisers have been designed to increase the efficiency of nebulisation. A jet nebuliser with a spacer attachment allows aerosol to pass into a holding chamber from which it is inhaled during inspiration, while expired air is diverted away from the chamber by a valve. In other systems the patient can manually control the input of compressed air into the nebuliser, allowing nebulisation to coincide with inspiration, or vents are added. 'Open vent' nebulisers allow shorter nebulisation time, whereas 'breath-assisted open vent' systems provide an increased amount of inspired drug.

A newer nebuliser is the adaptive aerosol delivery (AAD) system (Halolite), which delivers a precise dose of drug and then switches off (Figure 7.11). The device adapts to the patient's breathing pattern and delivers drug during inspiration only. It stops delivery when the required dose has been given.

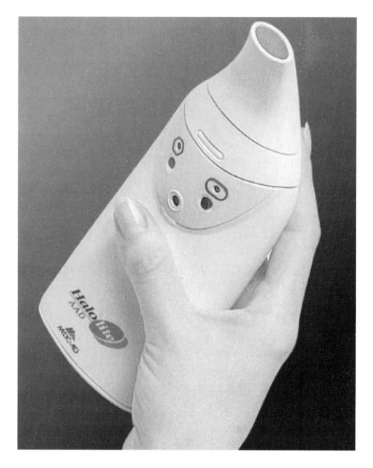

Figure 7.11 Halolite nebuliser. (Courtesy of Medic-Aid Ltd.)

Administration schedules

Nebulisers should be capable of generating a continuous cloud of fine drug particles. The patient should be advised to breathe normally through the mask or mouthpiece. The time required for the administration of an effective dose varies with the drug, its concentration in solution and the particle size distribution of the droplet spray. The period of administration must be balanced against the length of time that the patient is willing to sit and inhale the spray. It has been suggested that the optimum duration for continuous nebulisation is between five and ten minutes.

If dilution of nebuliser solutions is necessary, normal saline should be used to maintain isotonicity. Hypotonic solutions have been reported to aggravate respiratory symptoms through the production of bronchospasm.

Care of nebulisers

Many nebulising units are described as disposable. However, if they are used by one person and adequate care is taken in maintenance, a life of two to four months can be expected. Bacterial contamination of the aerosol and reservoir fluids in nebulisers used in the home is common if adequate hygienic measures are not taken. This can be a special problem if the solutions for nebulisation do not contain bacteriostatic agents.

Patients using nebulisers regularly should clean them daily; those using them intermittently should clean them after each use. The nebuliser, mask or mouthpiece should be disassembled, washed in warm water with a little detergent, and allowed to dry overnight. The nebuliser should be allowed to run with no drug in it before the next treatment.

Air filters on the nebuliser or the air compressor unit should also be changed regularly to minimise the risks of bacterial and fungal contamination. To prevent blockage of the capillary tube, drug solutions should ideally be removed from the unit after use. Blockage may occur through evaporation and crystallisation of the drug solution. Disposable components should be changed three to four times a year and compressors should be serviced annually.

Selection of a delivery device

The aerosol is delivered to the patient through a face mask or mouthpiece. Most patients can select the delivery device they prefer. For adults and older children, lung deposition is the same with mouthpiece and mask (provided the patient breathes through the mouth). Young children may be incapable of holding their lips tightly around a mouthpiece to achieve a good seal and the use of a mask may be preferable (although some children may be frightened by the occlusive nature of the mask). Face masks should be close fitting to the face.

For antibiotics, dornase alfa and steroids, mouthpieces should be used. For ipratropium, mouthpieces are preferrred to masks if there is a risk of glaucoma.

Purchase details

Nebulisers are not available on the NHS (apart from hand-operated atomisers, which are no longer used). Patients should not buy a nebuliser unless recommended to do so by their doctor.

A nebuliser system for domiciliary use can be purchased by the patient or family direct from a manufacturer. To confirm medical approval for its use, most manufacturers will only supply items to an individual on receipt of a letter from the patient's doctor. Items purchased in the UK are eligible for exemption from value-added tax (VAT) under Group 14 of Schedule 4 to the Finance Act of 1972.

Further reading

Royal Pharmaceutical Society of Great Britain (2000). *Practice Guidance on the Care of People with Asthma and Chronic Obstructive Pulmonary Disease.* London: Royal Pharmaceutical Society.

British Guidelines on Asthma Management 1995 review and position statement (1997). *Thorax* 52 Suppl 1: S1–21.

British Thoracic Society guidelines on current best practice for nebuliser treatment (1997). *Thorax* 52 Suppl 2: S1–106.

Cates CJ, Rowe BH (2001). Holding chambers versus nebulisers for beta-agonist treatment of acute asthma (Cochrane Review). In: The Cochrane Library 1. Oxford: Update Software.

National Institute for Clinical Excellence. Guidance on use of inhalers for under-5s. http://www.nice.org.uk

Inhaler devices for asthma (2000). *Drug Ther Bull* 38: 9–14.

Useful addresses

British Lung Foundation
78 Hatton Garden
London EC1N 8LD
Tel: 020 7831 5831
www.britishlungfoundation.co.uk

National Asthma Campaign
Providence House
Providence Place
London N1 0NT
Tel: 020 7226 2260
www.asthma.org.uk

National Asthma and Respiratory Training Centre
The Athenaeum
10 Church Street
Warwick CV34 4AB
Tel: 01926 493313
www.nartc.org.uk

Cystic Fibrosis Trust
11 London Road
Bromley
Kent BR1 1BY
Tel: 020 8464 7211
www.cftrust.org.uk

British Thoracic Society
6th floor, North Wing
New Garden House
78 Hatton Garden
London EC1N 8LD
Tel: 020 7831 8778
www.brit-thoracic.org.uk

8

Dietary products

Pamela Mason

This chapter reviews the diverse range of medical dietary products and the conditions for which they are indicated. Some special dietary treatments are initiated in hospital, but many of the conditions are not severely debilitating and the majority of patients may lead a relatively normal life at home. It is therefore probable that special foods will continue to be prescribed by the patient's GP and supplies obtained from the community pharmacy.

In the UK, the range of dietary products that may be supplied is covered by the guidelines issued by the Advisory Committee on Borderline Substances (ACBS).

The primary causes of conditions requiring special dietary manipulations may be broadly classified as:

- Intolerance
- Malabsorption
- Error(s) of metabolism.

This aetiological classification, however, is not exclusive (e.g. an intolerance condition can produce malabsorption, and an error of metabolism can give rise to intolerance). The classifications outlined below are based on the primary cause of the condition.

Other dietary modifications may be required for diseases that do not fall into the above three categories, and these are also discussed in this chapter. In each of the categories the products mentioned are those whose use for that condition is approved by the ACBS guidelines. The availability of items in the UK on National Health Service prescriptions, however, must be confirmed by reference to the current edition of the *Drug Tariff*.

Intolerance conditions

Carbohydrate

Lactose intolerance

Lactose ingested in the diet is broken down in the intestine to its constituent monosaccharides by the enzyme lactase (Figure 8.1).

The sole sources of lactose in the diet are human milk, which contains about 70 g/L, and cow's milk, which contains about 50 g/L. The enzyme lactase is specific for lactose and is found in the brush border cells of the intestine. These cells are continually undergoing regeneration and have a life of two to three days. In the absence of a challenge from lactose, the production of the enzyme decreases and eventually stops.

The enzyme deficiency may be:

- congenital: an inborn error of metabolism produces symptoms soon after birth
- primary (ethnic): lactase may disappear slowly between infancy and adulthood if there is no demand for it. Populations in which milk is not a part of the diet will therefore be lactase deficient. About 5% of white Europeans are lactase deficient; the proportion in the non-white population may be as high as 75%
- secondary: a temporary deficiency may occur after an intestinal infection.

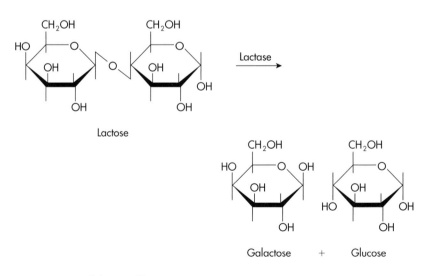

Figure 8.1 Breakdown of lactose.

The symptoms of a lack of the enzyme occur on ingestion of lactose and include intestinal discomfort, flatulence and watery diarrhoea. The symptoms are due to the increased osmotic pressure within the intestinal lumen caused by the presence of lactic acid and other products of fermentation. The diagnosis of lactose intolerance may be confirmed by a stool pH of less than 6 and a reducing-sugar concentration in urine of 0.5% or more when tested with Clinitest tablets.

The treatment of lactose intolerance involves the avoidance of all foods containing lactose (i.e. milk and milk products, and foods containing these ingredients). However, some patients with clinically proven lactose intolerance may be able to tolerate the small quantities of milk used to whiten tea and coffee. In young patients, the use of high-protein substitutes for milk products may prevent the development of symptoms. Examples of products which are lactose free are listed in Table 8.1.

Sucrose intolerance

An intolerance to sucrose in the diet is much less common than lactose intolerance. It develops mainly in children who have been weaned off breast milk and who are challenged with large quantities of sucrose, usually in the form of cane sugar.

The enzyme responsible for cleavage of the sucrose molecule is sucrase, present normally in intestinal brush border cells (Figure 8.2). Deficiency of the enzyme is inherited through an autosomal recessive

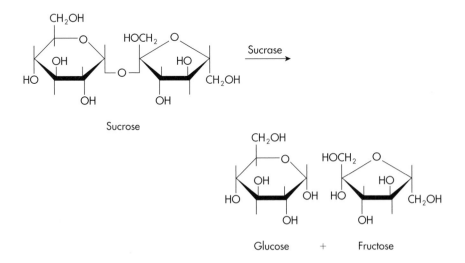

Figure 8.2 Breakdown of sucrose.

Table 8.1 Examples of products for carbohydrate intolerance

	Lactose intolerance	Lactose with sucrose intolerance	General disaccharide intolerance
AL 110	✓	–	–
Alfare	–	–	✓
Caloreen	–	–	✓
Calsip	–	–	✓
Comminuted chicken meat	✓	✓	–
Duocal Super Soluble and Liquid	–	–	✓
Enfamil Lactofree	✓	–	–
Farley's Soya Formula	✓	✓	–
Galactomin Formula 17	✓	✓	–
InfaSoy	✓	✓	–
Isomil Powder	✓	–	–
Maxijul LE, Liquid and Super Soluble	–	–	✓
Nutramigen	✓	✓	✓
Nutrison Soya	✓	–	✓
Pepdite	✓	–	✓
Pepti-Junior	–	✓	✓
Polycose Powder	–	–	✓
Pregestimil	✓	✓	✓
Prejomin	✓	✓	✓
Pro-Cal	–	–	✓
Prosobee	✓	✓	–
QuickCal	–	–	✓
SMA LF	✓	–	–
Vitajoule	–	–	✓
Vitasavoury	–	–	✓
Wysoy	✓	✓	–

✓ = items recommended.
– = items not recommended.

gene. The inability to deal with ingested sucrose may arise congenitally or as a consequence of other conditions (e.g. coeliac disease, see below).

Sucrose intolerance results in the presence of large quantities of undigested sucrose in the intestine. This generates gaseous abdominal distension and diarrhoea, with the frequent passage of watery stools. The avoidance of foods containing sucrose will eliminate the symptoms. Foods that contain significant quantities of sucrose include:

- All fruits except grapes, cherries (but not glacé cherries) and figs
- Fruit juice (except unsweetened tomato juice)

- All root vegetables, leeks, sweetcorn, and some canned vegetables
- Sugar-containing breakfast cereals
- Peas, beans (including baked beans) and lentils
- Sweetened bread, cakes, biscuits, pastries and pies
- Desserts and puddings, ice cream and jellies
- Jam, marmalade, syrup and treacle
- Sugar-containing drinks
- Drinking chocolate and malted milk drinks
- Canned or packet soups
- Gravy browning, pickles, chutneys and salad cream.

Foods that contain little or no sucrose and which may be acceptable include:

Meat	Fish	Tomatoes
Cheese	Eggs	Celery
Milk	Green salad and vegetables	Glucose
Butter	Unsweetened cereal and porridge	Fructose
Cream	Unsweetened breads	Some brands of honey

Items prescribable for sucrose intolerance under ACBS guidelines are listed in Table 8.1.

Protein/amino acid

Coeliac disease

An intolerance to gluten in the diet produces malabsorption of most nutrients from the gastrointestinal tract, owing to reversible changes in the mucous membranes of the upper ileum. Gluten is a protein and the term is used to describe the two components glutenin and gliadin. This pair of compounds is found in wheat, flour and other cereals (e.g. rye, oats and barley). It is not present in rice.

Until fairly recently, the incidence of coeliac disease (i.e. a reflection of the number of diagnosed cases) was quoted as 1 in 2500 and the prevalence (i.e. the number of people with the disease) as 1 in 1000. However, several screening studies have shown the prevalence to be far higher. In addition, the UK Coeliac Society has more than 32 000 registered members, but this may be only about half the total number of patients with coeliac disease in the UK. Moreover, coeliac disease was once regarded as a condition of childhood, but the number of newly diagnosed children is falling and the increased incidence is due to more frequent diagnosis in adults. The declining incidence in children is probably a result of better weaning practices and the fact that many commercially prepared weaning foods are gluten free. Adults are usually diagnosed between 30 and 40 years of age, but increasing numbers are diagnosed between 50 and 60 years of age, suggesting that the increased incidence reflects better diagnosis. Other conditions have been associated with coeliac disease (e.g. diabetes mellitus, lactose intolerance, infertility and autoimmune diseases).

Sensitivity to gluten produces intestinal atrophy, reducing the surface area available for absorption. In severe cases villi may be completely absent from the jejunum. Suggestions as to the cause of the sensitivity include idiosyncratic toxic reactions produced by gluten or an allergic reaction to its presence. The symptoms of gluten sensitivity are dominated by fatty diarrhoea, which is characterised by the passage of pale soft bulky stools which may also be foul-smelling. Other symptoms include, in young children, failure to thrive, retarded growth, a protruding stomach and periodic vomiting. In adults, other symptoms include loss of weight, chronic fatigue and failure to thrive.

Malabsorption results from the presence of intolerance. This may lead to anaemia (through effects on iron, folate and vitamin B_{12} absorption), rickets (through vitamin D malabsorption) and spontaneous haemorrhaging (caused by malabsorption of vitamin K). The severity of symptoms may fluctuate through life with unpredictable remissions and relapses. Antibody screening is the most sensitive method for detecting coeliac disease, but endoscopy and biopsy of intestinal tissue are required to confirm the diagnosis.

Most patients with coeliac disease will show a marked and maintained improvement in their condition if flour or cereals derived from wheat, rye and barley are eliminated from the diet. The role of oats is controversial. Many patients tolerate oats, but it is not clear whether they should definitely be recommended. Many experts still advise the exclusion of oats, partly because commercial oat products are frequently contaminated with wheat starch during the milling process. However, if the patient can tolerate uncontaminated oats, they offer a tremendous scope for improving the quality and variety of the diet. Corn, rice and potato flours are not harmful. Affected children may respond within weeks to the elimination of gluten from the diet. However, severely affected adults may take up to six months to show a sustained, positive improvement. Iron supplements and the administration of folic acid are usually required for the treatment of anaemia and mucous membrane disruptions (e.g. glossitis and stomatitis).

A major problem in selecting an appropriate balanced diet for patients with coeliac disease is the unadvertised use of gluten-containing wheat flour as a thickening agent, filler and 'carrier' for flavourings in a large number of proprietary foods. In an attempt to help patients to select an appropriate diet, the Coeliac Society was formed in 1968 and regularly publishes and updates a handbook of commercially available foods that are known to be gluten free.

A list of naturally occurring or manufactured foods which are gluten free is given in Table 8.2. Foods that contain gluten and which

Table 8.2 Naturally occurring or manufactured foods which are gluten free

Alcohol	Bought wines and spirits
Baking powder	Bicarbonate of soda, cream of tartar, tartaric acid, yeast (dried and fresh)
Beverages	Tea, 100% pure or instant coffee, bottled coffee, fizzy drinks, fruit juices, pure fruit cordials, Complan
Cereals	Arrowroot, buckwheat, maize, sweetcorn, rice, ground rice, sago, tapioca, soya, popcorn, Cornflakes, Frosties, Rice Krispies, Ricicles[a]
Cheeses	Plain, cheese, cottage cheese, cream cheese
Condiments/sauces	Salt, peppercorns, herbs, spices, essences
Fish	Fresh or canned in plain oil, plain frozen fish, cured fish, shellfish
Flour	Potato flour, rice flour, arrowroot, soya flour, cornflour
Fruits	Fresh, tinned or frozen fruits
Gelatin	Jellies and gelatin
Meat	Fresh meat, bacon, ham, poultry
Milk products	Milk (powdered, fresh and tinned), cream, butter, yoghurt (plain)
Eggs	
Nuts	All kinds of nuts
Oils	Lard, dripping, cooking oil, olive oil, margarine
Preserves	Jam, marmalade, honey, golden syrup, molasses, treacle
Vegetables and vegetable products	Plain, fresh or frozen, not in sauces, potatoes, plain potato crisps

[a] Some brands of breakfast cereals may contain malt extract as a flavouring agent. This may contain gluten.

should therefore be avoided are listed in Table 8.3. For the latest information, a copy of the current edition of the *Coeliac Handbook*, which may be purchased from the Coeliac Society, should be consulted.

A range of specially manufactured foods is available under ACBS guidelines for gluten-sensitive enteropathies (Table 8.4).

Dermatitis herpetiformis

Dermatitis herpetiformis is often regarded as a condition closely allied to coeliac disease, as it is an external manifestation of the disease. It is less common than coeliac disease: the prevalence is thought to be about 1 in 20 000, but this figure is under review. The presence of gluten contributes towards intensely irritating small blisters on pressure points over the body (e.g. elbows, buttocks and knees). Intestinal atrophy, similar to that seen in coeliac disease, may also occur. The skin condition significantly improves after the elimination of gluten from the diet, and management is therefore similar to that described for coeliac disease.

Treatment with dapsone (an agent used primarily in the treatment of leprosy) may improve the rash of dermatitis herpetiformis. However, when dapsone is used in isolation, the rash often returns when treatment is stopped.

If a strict gluten-free diet is adopted in conjunction with dapsone treatment, drug administration may usually be stopped after up to two years, beyond which relapses are infrequent. The gluten-free diet, however, must usually be continued indefinitely.

Table 8.3 Naturally occurring or manufactured foods which are *not* gluten free and should be avoided

---

Wheatflours; purchased bread, cakes or biscuits; crispbreads; crumbs made from wheat, rye, barley or oats; spaghetti, noodles and other pasta; semolina

Breakfast cereals made from wheat, rye, barley or oats (e.g. Weetabix, Wheatflakes, porridge oats, oatmeal, Ready Brek, All Bran, muesli)

Unprocessed bran

Suet

Barley-flavoured squashes

Communion wafers

Alcohol (beers may contain gluten-like substances)

Drinking chocolate from vending machines

Coated fried fish

Table 8.4 Items which have been approved by the Advisory Committee on Border-line Substances (ACBS) for gluten-sensitive enteropathies

Biscuits	Arnott gluten-free rice cookies
	Bi-Aglut gluten-free biscuits
	Glutafin biscuits (digestive, sweet [without chocolate or sultanas], tea)
	Glutano gluten-free biscuits
	Juvela digestive biscuits, savoury biscuits and tea biscuits
	Polial gluten-free biscuits
	Schar biscuits, savoy biscuits
Bread/bread mixes	Barkat gluten-free bread mix; brown or white rice bread (unsliced)
	Clara's Kitchen gluten-free bread mix; gluten-free high-fibre bread mix
	Dietary Specialities Mixes: brown or white bread, corn bread, white cake, white or fibre
	Ener-G brown and white rice bread, brown rice and maize bread, gluten-free tapioca bread, rice loaf
	Glutafin bread, multigrain white loaf (sliced or unsliced, white or parbaked), rolls (white or parbaked), fibre bread, mixes (white, multigrain white, fibre, multigrain fibre)
	Glutano wholemeal bread (sliced or parbaked), baguette, rolls (parbaked), white sliced bread (parbaked)
	Juvela gluten-free harvest mix; loaf and high-fibre loaf (sliced and unsliced), bread rolls, fibre bread rolls, parbaked rolls with or without fibre; mix; fibre mix
	Lifestyle gluten-free bread rolls, brown and white bread
	Pleniday bread loaf (sliced), country loaf (sliced), rustic loaf (parbaked baguette), petit pan
	Rite-dite gluten-free fibre rolls, high-fibre bread (sliced and unsliced), white bread (sliced and unsliced), white rolls
	Schar gluten-free bread, bread mix, bread rolls, cake mix, French bread (baguette), white bread buns, wholemeal bread
	Sunnyvale gluten-free bread
	Tritamyl brown bread mix, white bread mix
	Ultra gluten-free baguette, high-fibre bread
	Valpiform bread mix, country loaf, pastry mix, petites baguettes
Flour	Aproten gluten-free flour
	Glutano flour mix
	Orgran pizza and pastry mix
	Schar flour mix, wholemeal flour mix
	Tritamyl flour
	Trufree gluten-free flours

Table 8.4 Continued

Flour	No 1
	No 2 with rice bran
	No 3 for Cantabread
	No 4 white
	No 5 brown
	No 6 plain
	No 7 self-raising
	No 8 special dietary
Pasta	Bi-Aglut pasta (fusilli, macaroni, penne, spaghetti)
	Bi-Aglut lasagne
	Ener-G gluten-free rice pasta (cannelloni, lasagna, macaroni, shells, small shells, spaghetti, tagliatelli, vermicelli)
	Ener-G brown rice pasta (lasagna, macaroni, spaghetti)
	Glutafin pasta (lasagne, penne, spirals, spaghetti)
	Glutano pasta (animal shapes, macaroni, spaghetti, spirals, tagliatelle)
	Orgran pasta, lasagne (corn, rice and maize), shells (split pea and soya), spaghetti (buckwheat, corn, rice, rice and millet, rice and maize), spirals (organic brown rice)
	Pleniday pasta (penne rigate)
	Schar pasta (fusilli, lasagne, macaroni, pipette penne, rigatini, rings, shells, spaghetti)
	Tinkyada gluten-free brown rice pasta (elbows, fettucini, fusilli, penne, shells, spaghetti, spirals)
Pizza base	Barkat brown or white rice pizza crust
	Glutafin pizza base
	Juvela pizza bases
	Schar pizza base
	Ultra pizza base
Rusks/crackers	Bi-Aglut gluten-free crackers, cracker toast
	Glutafin crackers, high-fibre crackers
	Glutano crackers
	Juvela crispbread
	Schar cracker toast, crispbread
	Ultra cracker bread

Milk-protein sensitivity

The ability of a newborn baby to tolerate unfamiliar proteins may develop only slowly after birth. Cow's milk sensitivity, which occurs in up to 1% of all newborn babies, is a reaction to proteinaceous antigens (primarily β-lactoglobulin) present in milk.

Symptoms of milk-protein intolerance are usually absent when the baby is given mother's milk. They may develop during the first three months of life, suggesting a direct reaction to the challenge of unfamiliar proteins in cow's milk. Alternatively, they may appear after 6–18 months of life, indicating a defect in the response of the gastrointestinal wall to milk proteins.

Eczema and respiratory symptoms (e.g. wheeze, shortness of breath and recurrent colds) are classic signs of a chronic allergic reaction. The presence of persistent vomiting, diarrhoea and intestinal colic indicates gastrointestinal intolerance. Diarrhoea may be severe and accompanied by blood loss. The development of iron-deficiency anaemia is indicative of the baby's general failure to thrive.

Treatment consists of the replacement of cow's milk by a milk substitute (e.g. soya milk), following which symptoms usually recede within 24–48 hours. Continuation of substitution is usually recommended for up to 6–12 months before a rechallenge with cow's milk. At this stage most babies will tolerate the milk. Soya protein substitutes are most commonly used, although as many as one in four babies may also develop intolerance to this protein. If the intolerance is severe the avoidance of beef products may also be necessary, because of the presence of a similar range of proteins to that in cow's milk.

Products available under ACBS guidelines for the treatment of milk-protein intolerance are listed in Table 8.5.

Malabsorption conditions

Carbohydrate

Glucose/galactose malabsorption

Glucose/galactose malabsorption should be clearly differentiated from lactose intolerance (see above), in which a deficiency of the enzyme lactase prevents the breakdown of lactose to glucose and galactose. In the malabsorption condition, the disaccharidase enzyme is present and active. However, owing to a genetically determined deficiency in transport, glucose and galactose formed from the hydrolysis of lactose are not absorbed from the intestine. As a result, ingested lactose produces copious watery stools containing glucose and galactose. If malabsorption remains untreated, dehydration and lassitude may result, which may be fatal. Treatment consists of replacing lactose in the diet with fructose to provide an alternative carbohydrate source. Fructose does

Table 8.5 Products prescribable under ACBS guidelines for milk-protein intolerance

	Protein source	CHO	Protein	Fat
Comminuted chicken meat	Ground chicken meat	−	++++	−
Farley's Soya Formula	Soya	++++	++	+++
InfaSoy	Soya	++++	++	+++
Isomil Powder	Soya	+	+	+
Nutramigen	Casein	++++	++	++
Prosobee Powder	Soya	++++	++	+++
Wysoy	Soya	++++	++	+++

− none; + under 10%; ++ 10–19%; +++ 20–39%; ++++ 40–79%.

not produce diarrhoea but may generate a slow rise in blood glucose levels. Avoidance of foods containing lactose and a reduction in fat intake will reduce the severity of the diarrhoea. Dietary modifications must be maintained for life.

Protein/amino acid

Conditions in which protein/amino acid malabsorption occurs are due to an inability to absorb amino acids normally (e.g. Hartnup disease, cystinuria and 'blue diaper' syndrome) and to defects in pancreatic function, which affect protein digestion and absorption (e.g. cystic fibrosis).

Hartnup disease

In Hartnup disease, neutral amino acids (alanine, asparagine, citrulline, glutamine, histidine, isoleucine, leucine, phenylalanine, serine, threonine, tryptophan, tyrosine and valine) are not absorbed normally. Clinically, the lack of tryptophan absorption is the most important, producing a deficiency of nicotinamide. This deficiency results in a rash and peripheral neuritis normally associated with pellagra.

Cystinuria

In cystinuria, dibasic amino acids (lysine, arginine and ornithine) and cystine are absorbed in reduced quantities and renal excretion is greater than normal. Kidney stones form at an early age and life expectancy is greatly reduced owing to kidney damage.

'Blue diaper' syndrome

Reduced tryptophan absorption, followed by the excretion of large quantities of one of its metabolites, produces a blue colour in urine which stains nappies. Hypercalcaemia and calcium-induced kidney damage, rather than the effects of reduced tryptophan levels, produce the important clinical symptoms.

Cystic fibrosis

The most apparent clinical effects in cystic fibrosis are the thick, sticky and dry body secretions. These primarily affect the trachea and lungs, producing an environment ripe for bacterial infections. Pancreatic secretions are also affected, becoming viscous and sticky. The pancreatic duct becomes blocked, preventing the release of pancreatic enzymes. As a result, the digestion of proteins and fats is severely impaired (for a more detailed description of cystic fibrosis, see Chapter 7).

Malabsorption of proteins causes muscle wasting, and excess intestinal fat produces steatorrhoea.

Fat

Intestinal lymphangiectasia

In intestinal lymphangiectasia the lymphatic drainage channels are not properly developed. This leads to an absence of lymph fluid, which results in fat malabsorption.

Replacing long-chain triglycerides with medium-chain triglycerides (MCT) (which are better absorbed than the longer-chain fats) provides adequate fat material.

Nutritional deficiencies produced by malabsorption must be overcome by the use of appropriate dietary supplements. In order for treatment to be successful, however, the underlying cause of the malabsorption condition must also be treated. A list of products that may be used for the treatment of all types of malabsorption is given in Table 8.6.

Table 8.6 Treatment of malabsorption conditions

Nutritionally complete feeds
Caprilon Formula
Complan Ready-to-Drink
Elemental 028 and Elemental 028 Extra
Emsogen
Enrich
Ensure and Ensure Powder
Frebini
Fresubin Energy and Fresubin Energy Fibre
Fresubin 1000 and Fresubin 2000
Infatrini
Isosource Energy, Fibre and Standard
Jevity
MCT Pepdite
Novasource GI Control
Nutrini Standard
Nutrison Multi-fibre, Pepti Liquid, Soya and Standard
Nutrodrip Energy, Fibre and Standard
Osmolite Liquid and Plus
Paediasure Liquid, Liquid with fibre and Plus
Pepdite
Peptamen
Pepti-Junior
Pregestimil
SMA High Energy
Sondalis Fibres, ISO Junior and 1.5

Nutritional supplements
Clinutren Dessert, ISO and 1.5
Enlive
Enrich Plus
Ensure Bar and Plus
Formance
Forticreme
Fortifresh
Fortijuice
Fortimel
Fortisip and Fortisip Multi-Fibre
Fresubin 750 MCT
Nutrison Energy, MCT and Pepti Powder
Perative
Protein Forte
Provide Xtra
Resource Shake and Benefiber
Survimed OPD

Table 8.6 Continued

Minerals
Aminogram Mineral Mixture
Metabolic Mineral Mixture

Protein supplements
Caprilon Formula
Comminuted Chicken Formula
Duocal Super Soluble and Liquid
Maxipro Super Soluble
MCT Pepdite
Neocate and Neocate Advance
Pepdite

Fat sources
Alembicol D
Calogen
Caprilon Formula
Liquigen
MCT Pepdite
Medium chain triglyceride oil
Pro-Cal
QuickCal
Vitasavoury

Carbohydrate sources
Caloreen
Calsip
Hycal
Maxijul LE, Liquid and Super Soluble
Novasource GI control
Polycal Powder and Liquid
Polycose
Pro-Cal
QuickCal
Resource Benefiber
Vitajoule
Vitasavoury

Fat/carbohydrate sources
Calshake
Duobar
Duocal Liquid and Super Soluble
Scandishake

Errors of metabolism

Carbohydrate

Galactosaemia

The main source of galactose in the diet is the cleavage of lactose present in milk (see above). After absorption from the intestine, galactose is metabolised to glucose through a series of reactions, one of which is by the action of glucose 1-phosphate uridyl transferase, an enzyme normally present in the liver from birth. In galactosaemia the activity of this enzyme is diminished, which leads to the accumulation of galactose in tissues. An alternative metabolic pathway via the reductase enzyme to galactitol (dulcitol) is followed.

Galactitol and galactose accumulate in diverse tissues (e.g. nerve endings and kidney tissue). The lens of the eye stores galactitol, giving rise to a high incidence of cataracts. If the condition remains untreated, young children may become mentally retarded. Liver damage, producing vomiting and diarrhoea, may also occur.

Galactokinase deficiency

The initial step in the conversion of galactose to glucose is its phosphorylation, a reaction mediated by the enzyme galactokinase. The absence of this enzyme produces symptoms similar to those of galactosaemia, although galactokinase deficiency is much less common than galactosaemia.

Irrespective of the enzyme defect, the treatment of galactosaemia and galactokinase deficiency is directed towards the reduction of galactose intake. As lactose is the primary source of galactose, a lactose-free diet will alleviate or prevent the symptoms. It should be noted, however, that the ACBS recommendations do not include all dietary products deemed suitable for lactose intolerance. A lactose-free diet must normally be maintained for life. Items approved for galactosaemia and galactokinase deficiency under ACBS guidelines are listed in Table 8.7.

Glycogen storage diseases

This all-encompassing description applies to several variants of autosomal recessive biochemical disorders in which the conversion of glycogen to glucose in the liver is impaired or unable to take place (Figure 8.3). The most common disorders are due to glucose 6-phosphatase

Table 8.7 Items approved by ACBS guidelines for galactosaemia/galactokinase deficiency

ALL 110
Farley's Soya Formula
Galactomin Formula 17
InfaSoy
Isomil Powder
Prosobee
Wysoy

deficiency (type 1 glycogen storage disease). Glucose 6-phosphatase removes the phosphate group from glucose 6-phosphate to produce free glucose. Distribution of the enzyme is restricted to the liver. Muscle and brain both lack the enzyme and the ability to produce glucose in this way.

The absence of glucose 6-phosphatase prevents the conversion of glycogen to glucose, which normally occurs in response to an increased demand for glucose. Hypoglycaemia may occur when the body's energy requirements increase, and is often identified in early childhood. Other symptoms include a failure to thrive, abdominal distension and diarrhoea. Children who present with this condition at an older age are often of short stature and have signs of hepatomegaly. If the condition remains untreated, growth may be slow and adult stature may be considerably reduced. Gout and benign hepatic tumours are other complications in adult patients.

Hypoglycaemia is treated by regular ingestion of glucose throughout the day. Uncooked corn starch, which may act as a source of sustained-release glucose, may be suitable for older children.

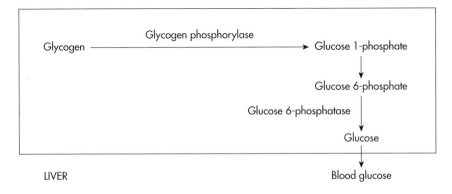

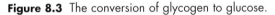

Figure 8.3 The conversion of glycogen to glucose.

Glycogen phosphorylase deficiency is a less common variant, but the net result is the same as in glucose 6-phosphatase deficiency. The absence of the enzyme prevents the removal of glucose monomers from the glycogen polymer.

High-carbohydrate low-protein diets must be taken regularly to provide a steady level of blood glucose. High-carbohydrate products available for glycogen storage diseases and approved under ACBS guidelines are described in Table 8.8.

Functional and ketotic hypoglycaemia

Functional hypoglycaemia is caused by excess insulin production or decreased breakdown of insulin. This may greatly reduce blood sugar levels two to four hours after a meal.

Ketotic hypoglycaemia occurs mainly in children between one and five years of age. It is due to the impaired release of glucogenic and ketogenic amino acids (e.g. leucine, phenylalanine and tyrosine) from muscle tissue.

Ketone bodies are found in the urine immediately before hypoglycaemia becomes evident. Intake should be modified to provide a high-carbohydrate low-protein diet that also minimises fat intake.

Items recommended for hypoglycaemia under the ACBS guidelines are listed in Table 8.8.

Table 8.8 Items approved by ACBS guidelines for glycogen storage diseases and hypoglycaemia

	Glycogen storage disease	*Hypoglycaemia*
Caloreen	✓	✓
Corn Flour	✓	✓
Corn Starch	✓	✓
Glucose	✓	–
Maxijul LE	✓	✓
Maxijul Liquid (orange)	✓	✓
Maxijul Super Soluble	✓	✓
Polycal	✓	✓
Polycose	✓	✓
Pro-Cal	✓	✓
QuickCal	✓	✓
Vitajoule	✓	✓
Vitasavoury	✓	✓

Protein/amino acid

Phenylketonuria

The main source of phenylalanine in the infant diet is breast milk. In normal metabolism, phenylalanine is converted by a specific hydroxylase enzyme into tyrosine (Figure 8.4). In phenylketonuria (PKU), genetic defects in the production of the enzyme mean that this conversion does not take place. Instead, phenylalanine is metabolised via a transaminase reaction to phenylpyruvic acid (a phenylketone). Further metabolism to phenyllactic acid and phenylacetic acid occurs subsequently (Figure 8.5).

The enzyme deficiency has an incidence of about 1 in 20 000. It is the most common inborn error of metabolism and was the first found to respond to dietary modifications.

Symptoms are due to an accumulation of phenylalanine in blood, urine and tissues. This produces retardation of CNS development, overactivity and epileptic seizures. Parents may become aware of unresponsiveness and delays in developmental milestones. Symptoms may also be caused by a deficiency of tyrosine. The consequent lack of melanin pigmentation produces fair hair, pale skin and blue eyes. If the condition is identified at or soon after birth and appropriate treatment is undertaken, CNS development may be normal. Total population screening for PKU is therefore carried out soon after birth, using the Guthrie bacterial inhibition test.

A diet low in, but not totally excluding, phenylalanine is required. Dietary intake must include small quantities of phenylalanine for tissue growth and repair. In babies, milk products which are low in phenylalanine must be substituted for mother's or cow's milk, although such preparations must be high in calories. Amino acid supplements lacking in phenylalanine must also be given. Preparations containing protein

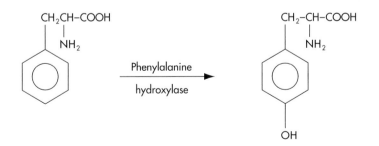

Figure 8.4 The conversion of phenylalanine to tyrosine.

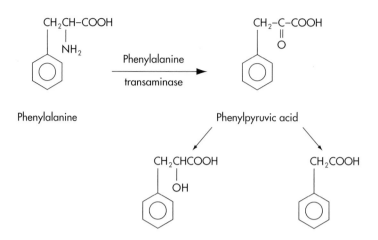

Figure 8.5 The metabolism of phenylalanine in phenylketonuria.

hydrolysates are almost nutritionally complete and may be particularly suited to infants.

After weaning, the provision of an adequate diet becomes more complicated. Foods with minimal phenylalanine content (e.g. sugar, jams, and vegetable and cooking oils) may be used with impunity. Fruit and vegetables also contain only small quantities of the amino acid and may be taken in normal amounts on their own or in stews, salads and sauces. Lists of quantities of foods containing the equivalent of 50 mg phenylalanine are available from the National Society of Phenylketonuria and Allied Disorders (see below).

For older children, protein-rich foods (e.g. meat, fish, eggs and cheese) should be taken only in limited quantities. The minimum requirements for phenylalanine may be provided by giving measured amounts of cereals, milk, vegetables and fruit, together with low-phenylalanine bread. Mineral and vitamin supplements may also be required, and a carefully formulated diet is usually arranged by the hospital dietitian.

Until recently the approach was that, once the brain had reached its maximum development, rigid adherence to a low-phenylalanine diet might no longer be necessary. This stage is generally considered to have been reached by eight to ten years of age. However, relaxation of the diet and high blood levels of phenylalanine can lead to a reduction in IQ, learning disabilities and behavioral disturbances in children and adolescents. This has led to the suggestion that the diet should be restricted throughout life. Lifelong dietary restriction is a difficult issue and clear evidence for overwhelming benefit is lacking. However, some experts advocate lifelong dietary restriction of phenylalanine, whereas others maintain that, after a full and informed discussion, the patient should decide. Whatever the patient decides, a full annual review is necessary.

Women with PKU who wish to start a family should be seen at a clinic where there are experts on PKU. Strict dietary control is necessary before conception and throughout pregnancy to minimise the risks of congenital abnormalities (e.g. mental retardation, microcephaly and congenital heart disease).

Foods and dietary supplements available for the treatment of phenylketonuria are listed in Table 8.9.

Table 8.9 Products approved by ACBS guidelines for the treatment of phenylketonuria

Foods	
Biscuits	Aminex low-protein biscuits, cookies and rusks Aproten biscuits dp low-protein butterscotch-flavoured or chocolate-flavoured chip cookies Juvela low-protein cookies (chocolate chip, orange and cinnamon flavour) Loprofin low-protein sweet biscuits, chocolate cream-filled biscuits, cookies (chocolate chip, cinnamon), wafers (orange, chocolate, vanilla) Ultra PKU biscuits, cookies, savoy biscuits Valpiform shortbread biscuits
Bread	Juvela low-protein loaf (sliced and unsliced), bread rolls Loprofin low-protein bread (sliced and unsliced), bread (canned, with or without salt), fibre bread (sliced and unsliced) Ultra low-protein, canned white bread Ultra PKU bread
Crispbread	Aproten crispbread Loprofin low-protein crackers
Egg replacer	Energen low-protein egg replacer Loprofin egg replacer
Flour	Ultra PKU flour
Mixes	Aproten bread mix, cake mix Juvela low-protein mix Loprofin low-protein mix Rite Diet low-protein baking mix, flour mix
Pizza bases	Ultra PKU pizza base

Table 8.9 Continued

Pasta	Aproten annelini, ditalini, rigatini, spaghetti, tagliatelle
	Loprofin low-protein pasta (macaroni, penne, spaghetti long, pasta, spirals, vermicelli)
	Promin low-protein pasta (alphabets, macaroni, shells, shortcut spaghetti, spirals), pasta tricolour (alphabets, shells, spirals), pasta meal
Rice	Aglutella low-protein rice
	Promin pasta imitation rice
Supplements	Aminogran Food Supplement (powder and tablets)
	Aminogran Mineral Mixture
	Analog LCP
	Analog XP
	Lofenalac
	Loprofin PKU Drink
	Metabolic Mineral Mixture
	Milupa PKU2 and PKU3
	Phlexy-10 exchange system
	Phelexyvits
	PK Aid 4
	PKU-gel
	Sno-Pro
	L-Tyrosine Supplement
	XP Maxamaid
	XP Maxamum

Homocystinuria

Homocystinuria (HCU) is the second most common amino acid metabolic disorder after phenylketonuria, and is due to a deficiency of the liver enzyme cystathionine synthetase.

In methionine metabolism, homocysteine is normally converted by cystathionine synthetase to cystathionine, an amino acid which is subsequently used in the synthesis of cysteine. In the absence of cystathionine synthetase, homocysteine is instead converted to homocystine (Figure 8.6).

Homocystine, which is not normally found in body fluids, is excreted in the urine. Its presence is detected by reaction with sodium cyanide and sodium nitroprusside solutions, a positive result producing a deep red colour.

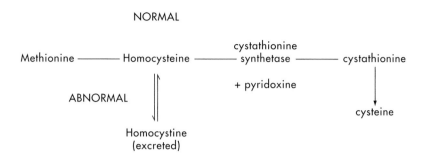

Figure 8.6 The metabolism of homocysteine.

Pyridoxine (vitamin B_6) is a cofactor in the conversion of homocysteine to cystathionine. In some patients, treatment with large doses of pyridoxine may produce a clinical improvement.

The presence of homocystine produces mental retardation in about half of the patients who have a deficiency of cystathionine synthetase. Paradoxically, the rest may show normal or nearly normal intelligence. Mental deficiency has also been linked to decreased body levels of cysteine, as this amino acid is converted to taurine, a putative neurotransmitter.

Other clinical signs of homocystinuria include elongated long bones that are susceptible to fracture owing to defects in calcification. Lens dislocation in the eye is a further indication of abnormal collagen synthesis.

Treatment is directed towards limiting the dietary intake of methionine to reduce the levels of homocystine in body tissues. Increased intake of cysteine must also take place to compensate for the reduced levels produced by the enzyme deficiency. Products available under ACBS guidelines are:

- Analog Xmet
- Methionine-Free Amino Acid Mix
- X Met Maxamaid
- X Met Maxamum.

Maple-syrup urine disease

Maple-syrup urine disease (branched-chain ketoaciduria) is a potentially fatal metabolic disorder whose name derives from the sweet, caramel-like smell of the urine which has been likened to that of maple syrup.

The disease is caused by a block in the catabolism of three branched-chain amino acids. This leads to increased levels of the oxoacid derivatives of the amino acids in body fluids and cells (e.g. urine, blood cells and cerebrospinal fluid), with leucine levels commonly predominating (Figure 8.7).

Accumulation of these catabolic byproducts results in drastic changes in body activities, primarily through effects on brain metabolism. The formation of normal synaptic intracellular connections is severely impaired, leading to either death or significant mental retardation.

Treatment consists of limiting the intake of the three branched-chain amino acids to the body's minimal requirements. Management may sometimes be possible by restricting only the most seriously elevated amino acid, usually leucine. If the child survives, a low-protein diet based on sugar, fruits, gluten-free flour, and gelatin is required. Products available under ACBS guidelines are:

- Analog MSUD
- MSUD Maxamaid
- MSUD Maxamum
- MSUD Aid III.

Histidinaemia

Histidine is used in the synthesis of protein and the formation of histamine, carnosine and homocarnosine. It is normally metabolised to urocanic acid by the action of histidine-deaminase (histidase).

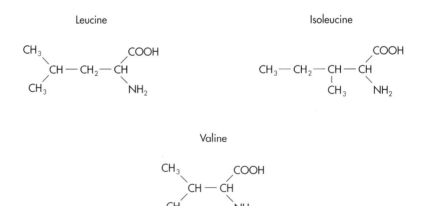

Figure 8.7 The metabolic pathway in maple-syrup urine disease.

In histidinaemia, lack of the hepatic enzyme produces large quantities of histidine in the blood. Histidine is also metabolised via an alternative metabolic pathway to imidazole pyruvic acid. Delayed development, both physical and mental, and speech disorders are the most common symptoms.

Restriction of histidine intake is the only effective treatment. However, in young children retarded growth may result from this restriction.

There is no specific product available for histidinaemia under the ACBS guidelines. Low-protein products are usually prescribed.

Glutaric aciduria

Glutaric aciduria is a disorder of lysine and tryptophan metabolism in which a deficiency of the enzyme glutaryl-CoA dehydrogenase results in elevated levels and increased excretion of glutaric acid. The condition develops during the first years of life, most patients dying within the first 10 years. Symptoms include mental retardation and spasticity.

There is one product available for glutaric aciduria under the ACBS guidelines: X Lys Low Try Maxamaid.

Hyperlysinaemia

Characterised by an excess of lysine in the blood, this is an autosomal recessive aminoacidopathy caused by deficiency of an enzyme involved in lysine metabolism. The condition has been linked to congenital mental retardation, but this association is not proven.

There are two products available for hyperlysinaemia under ACBS guidelines: Analog X Lys and X Lys Maxamaid.

Hypermethioninaemia

Hypermethionaemia is a disorder of sulphur amino acid metabolism, in which a deficiency of the enzyme methionine adenosyltransferase prevents the synthesis of S-adenosylmethionine from methionine. This leads to elevated levels of methionine. It is treated by a low-protein diet, and the following products are available under ACBS guidelines:

- Analog X Met
- Methionine Free Amino Acid Mix
- X Met Maxamaid
- X Met Maxamum.

Isovaleric acidaemia

Isovaleric acidaemia has an incidence of less than 1 in 200 000 and is a disorder of branched-chain amino acid metabolism in which there is a deficiency of the enzyme isovaleryl-CoA dehydrogenase. This results in failure to convert isovaleryl-CoA to 3-methylcrotonyl CoA, one of the intermediate substances in the metabolism of leucine. Isovaleric acid is excreted, giving the urine a pungent odour of sweaty feet. Other symptoms include lethargy progressing to coma, vomiting, and an aversion to protein-rich food. The condition is treated by a diet low in protein and/or leucine, and the following products are available under ACBS guidelines:

- Leucine-Free Amino Acid Mix
- X Leu Analog
- X Leu Maxamaid.

Methylmalonic acidaemia

This is a disorder in which there may be a deficiency of the apo enzyme methylmalonyl-CoA mutase or a defect in the synthesis of the cofactor adenosyl cobalamin. In some of the latter patients homocystinaemia occurs as well as methylmalonic acidaemia. This is due to defective synthesis of methylcobalamin as well as adenosyl cobalamin, the former being a cofactor for one of the reactions catalysing the remethylation of homocysteine to methionine.

The most severely affected patients have no functional mutase enzyme and suffer a severe illness during the neonatal period with grunting respiration, vomiting, dehydration and drowsiness. Metabolic acidosis and ketosis develop, leading to coma and death. Other patients have a structurally altered mutase, and may respond to dietary protein restriction. Patients with combined methylmalonic acidaemia and homocystinaemia are biochemically and genetically distinct. Their symptoms include failure to thrive, lethargy, poor feeding, developmental retardation and megaloblastic anaemia.

Products available for the treatment of this condition under ACBS guidelines include:

- Analog X Met, Thre Val, Isoleu
- X Met, Thre, Val, Isoleu Maxamaid
- X Met, Thre, Val, Isoleu Maxamum
- Methionine, Threonine, Valine-Free and Isoleucine-Low Amino Acid Mix.

Propionic acidaemia

This is a disorder with an incidence of 1 in 100 000 in which there is a deficiency of the enzyme propionyl-CoA carboxylase. This leads to metabolic acidosis and ketosis; sometimes hypoglycaemia may be present. Symptoms include developmental retardation, hypotonia, lethargy, episodic vomiting and intolerance to protein. There is heterogeneity in the severity and age of onset, with later-onset patients responding better to treatment.

Treatment involves a low protein intake with restriction of isoleucine, valine, methionine and threonine. Products available for the treatment of this condition under ACBS guidelines include:

- Analog X Met, Thre,Val, Isleu
- X Met, Thre, Val, Isoleu Maxamaid
- X Met, Thre Val, Isoleu Maxamum
- Methionine, Threonine, Valine-Free, Isoleucine-Low Amino Acid Mix.

Tyrosinaemia

Tyrosinaemia, of which there are several forms, arises as a result of a defect in tyrosine metabolism. Type 1 is due to a deficiency of fumaryl acetoacetase. Acute and chronic forms exist, with the former developing during the first few months of life; symptoms include a cabbage-like odour and death from liver failure in infancy. The chronic type is characterised by chronic liver disease, renal tubular dysfunction, hypophosphataemic rickets, and death in childhood. Type 2 occurs as a result of hepatic tyrosine transaminase deficiency and is marked by the crystallisation of accumulated tyrosine in the epidermis and cornea, and frequently by mental retardation.

Dietary treatment involves restriction of phenylalanine, tyrosine, and possibly methionine. Products available for this condition under ACBS guidelines are:

- Analog X Phen, Tyr; Analog X Phen, Tyr, Met
- X Phen, Tyr, Maxamaid
- XPTM Tyrosidon
- XPT Tyrosidon.

Fat

Hyperlipidaemias (hyperlipoproteinaemias)

Hyperlipidaemia is the presence in the blood of abnormally high concentrations of lipids (i.e. cholesterol and triglycerides) or lipoproteins. Lipids are insoluble in water and are therefore transported round the body bound to various lipoproteins. These include chylomicrons, which carry dietary triglyceride from the intestine into the blood; very low-density lipoproteins (VLDL), which are synthesised in the liver and transport triglycerides made in the liver to other tissues; low-density lipoproteins (LDL), which transport cholesterol from the liver to the tissues; and high-density lipoproteins (HDL), which transport excess cholesterol from the tissues to the liver for excretion in the bile.

High levels of LDL and VLDL are considered to be risk factors for coronary heart disease and high levels of HDL to be protective, although research is now identifying the importance of other lipoprotein risk factors.

There are various types of hyperlipidaemia, some of which are inherited (familial hyperlipidaemias). Although there are similarities in treatment, familial hyperlipidaemias should be distinguished from raised blood cholesterol levels, which may occur as a result of obesity and/or poor diet. In the genetic hyperlipidaemias the concentration of lipids can be extremely high, which may be due to excessive synthesis in the liver, or to reduced conversion of cholesterol to bile acids and steroids.

Dietary treatment of familial hyperlipidaemias depends on the type, but usually involves fat restriction.

Type 1 hyperlipoproteinaemia is caused by an absence of the enzyme lipoprotein lipase. This enzyme is responsible for the hydrolysis of chlyomicrons in the adipose tissue. Its absence means that chylomicrons stay in the circulation for long periods (more than 14 hours after a period of starvation) and triglycerides are deposited in tissue.

Hyperlipoproteinaemia commonly occurs in young children, producing severe abdominal pain and the deposition of cholesterol in the skin, corneas and blood vessels.

Patients may be treated by restricting dietary fat and replacing long-chain (C12–C20) triglycerides with medium-chain (C6–C12) triglycerides to reduce lipoprotein plasma levels. Medium-chain triglycerides are also more easily hydrolysed and absorbed from the intestine than the long-chain compounds normally found in fat. Products available under the ACBS guidelines for the treatment of hyperlipoproteinaemia (type 1) are Alembicol D, Liquigen and MCT Oil (medium-chain triglyceride oil).

Long-chain acyl-CoA dehydrogenase deficiency

This is a disorder of fatty acid metabolism leading to metabolic acidosis and hypoglycaemia. Symptoms include, after fasting, recurrent coma and recurrent vomiting. Treatment involves avoidance of fasting, a high carbohydrate intake and a low intake of long-chain fatty acids. The one product available under ACBS guidelines for this condition is Monogen.

Carnitine palmitoyl transferase deficiency

Carnitine palmitoyl transferase catalyses the transfer of long-chain fatty acids between coenzyme A and carnitine and is therefore involved in lipid metabolism. In this disorder the enzyme is abnormally regulated, resulting in muscle ache, fatigue and myoglobinuria, but without the accumulation of lipids. It is an autosomal recessive trait and has a lower incidence in women than in men. The one product available under ACBS guidelines for this condition is Monogen.

Refsum's disease

This condition arises as a result of a deficiency of phytanic acid α-hydroxylase, leading to elevated levels of phytanic acid. Symptoms may include cerebellar ataxia, ichthyosis, retinitis pigmentosa and nerve deafness. Skeletal abnormalities may also be present. Dietary treatment involves the elimination of dairy produce, which is a source of phytanic acid.

Fresubin Liquid and Sip Feeds are available under ACBS guidelines for the treatment of this condition.

Other dietary modifications

Liver disease

The term 'chronic liver disease' encompasses a range of conditions for which dietary management is as varied as the aetiology. Conditions range from hepatic portal hypertension and obstructive jaundice to cirrhosis and hepatic encephalopathy. Dietary management is necessary to provide low-protein high-carbohydrate diets, with the occasional use of high-fat diets to provide a concentrated form of energy in nutritionally depleted patients.

The liver fulfils a wide variety of nutritional and metabolic functions. These include acting as a storage reservoir for iron, vitamins and glycogen, and the metabolism of fats (to lipoproteins and bile acids), carbohydrates (glucose to glycogen and vice versa) and proteins (amino acids to plasma proteins and urea). The liver also converts excess dietary proteins to glucose (gluconeogenesis) and excretes cholesterol and other steroids.

Damage to liver cells (hepatocytes) is produced by acute and chronic disease. Chronic liver disease and cirrhosis may cause damage through deposition of fibrous material. Common causes of liver damage (particularly in the western world) are infective agents (e.g. hepatitis A and hepatitis B viruses), excessive consumption of alcohol, drug administration and an inadequate diet (primarily lack of protein and vitamin B). Conversely, excessive circulating levels of fat (e.g. caused through overeating or uncontrolled diabetes) may also lead to fatty changes in the liver.

Acute liver disease

Acute hepatitis (e.g. after viral infection) requires no specific dietary treatment. However, if there is marked jaundice, reduced levels of bile salts may lead to decreased gastrointestinal absorption of fat. It may be necessary to restrict dietary intake of fat and ensure adequate or increased carbohydrate intake to satisfy energy requirements.

Chronic liver disease

Alcoholism is a common cause of chronic hepatitis and cirrhosis. Although no specific dietary treatment may be necessary, many alcoholics are chronically malnourished and may need advice on changing and improving dietary intake once their addiction has been successfully treated. Malnourishment may also be a characteristic of patients with cirrhosis. High-energy high-protein diets are required to correct malnourishment, although a high intake of protein may precipitate hepatic encephalopathy (see below). Medium-chain (C8–C10) triglycerides may be necessary in the presence of low dietary fat tolerance.

Ascites

The accumulation of large quantities of sodium-rich fluid in the peritoneal cavity may be a consequence of portal hypertension and reduced synthesis of plasma proteins (especially albumin). A high-protein low-sodium diet may be necessary to treat ascites, in conjunction with the administration of diuretics.

Hepatic encephalopathy

The liver is unable to metabolise protein (particularly aromatic amino acids) in excess of dietary requirements. As a result, aromatic amino acids may accumulate in the plasma. The action of intestinal bacteria on the excess protein leads to the production of ammonia, which is normally detoxified by the liver through its conversion to urea. In the presence of decreased liver function, the build-up of ammonia levels in the plasma causes hepatic encephalopathy through the entry of ammonia into the brain. As a result, normal brain function is impaired.

In severe hepatic encephalopathy initial therapy includes severe restriction of protein from the diet, but the level of restriction varies. At the earliest signs of recovery from liver failure, diets which are low, rather than totally lacking, in protein are indicated. A small amount of protein must be taken in the diet to prevent depletion of body stores by the normal turnover. Low-protein products (some of which are also gluten free and are used in the treatment of coeliac disease) provide a range of foods for dietary management (Table 8.10).

A high intake of carbohydrate is protein sparing and may also aid in the recovery of damaged liver cells. Fat sources prescribable for chronic liver disease and cirrhosis provide a concentrated energy source. These products, however, are not suitable as a sole nutritional source in liver disease (Table 8.10).

Renal disease

In renal disease the maintenance of normal tissue and fluid levels of nutrients and electrolytes (homoeostasis) is impaired. Dietary measures in the treatment of renal disease are complicated by differences in the predominant effects.

In generalised disease, simple measures to prevent the accumulation of materials in the body include reducing fluid and electrolyte intake to the minimum required to sustain life. Reducing the intake of protein may also be beneficial, by minimising the production of urea.

Dietary intake of sodium may require restriction in diseases in which excretory function is impaired (e.g. nephrotic syndrome). Conversely, tubular disease leads to the loss of excessive quantities of

Table 8.10 Total feeds

Complan Ready-to-Drink
Elemental 028
Emsogen
Enrich
Ensure Liquid and Powder
Frebini
Fresubin Energy
Fresubin Energy Fibre Tube Feed and Liquid
Fresubin 1000 and 1200 Complete
Fresubin Original Fibre
Infatrini
Isosource Energy, Fibre and Standard
Jevity, Jevity Plus
Novasource GI control
Nutrini Extra, Fibre and Standard
Nutrison Multi Fibre, Soya and Standard
Osmolite and Osmolite Plus
Paediasure Liquid, Liquid with fibre
Paediasure Plus
Peptamen
Peptisorb
Sondalis Fibre, ISO and 1.5
Sondalis Junior

All preparations except Infatrini are contraindicated in infants under 12 months of age.
All products except Paediasure and Sondalis Junior should be used with caution between one and five years of age.

electrolytes (especially sodium) and water, and losses must be replaced by an appropriate increase in dietary intake.

Dietary management is considered a conservative form of treatment and may be used while the patient is awaiting dialysis or transplantation. Haemodialysis and peritoneal dialysis (see Chapter 11) may also demand dietary management (see below).

Acute renal failure

Acute renal failure is a sudden failure of kidney function owing to poor glomerular filtration. This condition may be precipitated by a sudden fall in blood pressure (caused by shock, haemorrhage or burns), glomerulonephritis and pyelonephritis (see Chapter 11). During the early stages of the condition urine output is absent or severely reduced. Protein restriction, in conjunction with the protein-sparing administration of glucose or glucose polymers, may be temporarily instituted, but only in patients who are non-catabolic. A high-protein diet will be required in patients who are catabolic. Potassium supplements may be necessary, and as renal function improves a staged return to a normal diet may be possible.

Chronic renal failure

Chronic renal failure occurs over a longer period than the acute condition and develops gradually and insidiously (see Chapter 11). The role of diet in slowing the progression of this condition is controversial. Decreased protein intake is sometimes advocated to reduce urea production and alleviate symptoms of anorexia and vomiting. An added advantage of the restriction of dietary protein is the reduction in phosphate intake. Decreased phosphate levels are necessary to prevent further kidney damage through the precipitation of calcium phosphate around the tubules.

Other dietary modifications include the intake of large quantities of carbohydrate to satisfy energy requirements and to reduce hunger. Sodium restriction may be necessary to prevent the harmful effects of hypertension on kidney function, and to limit the production of oedema in the peripheral tissues and in the lungs.

Haemodialysis

For patients undergoing haemodialysis, increased protein intake (compared to the pre-dialysis state) is necessary to replace amino acids lost during dialysis. Potassium and phosphate restrictions are required, and blood pressure and thirst are controlled by limiting sodium intake. Fluid restriction is also essential, as most patients produce no urine.

Peritoneal dialysis

In patients undergoing peritoneal dialysis sodium and fluid restrictions must be adopted to limit fluid overload caused by the absorption of large quantities of glucose through the peritoneum. Oral ingestion of carbohydrates must also be restricted to prevent obesity and hyperlipidaemia. Some protein is invariably lost through the peritoneum in normal dialysis, and the quantity increases dramatically in the presence of peritonitis. Protein supplements may therefore be needed by patients undergoing peritoneal dialysis.

A complete list of products that can be used in the treatment of renal disease is given in Table 8.11.

Table 8.11 Low-protein diets for chronic liver disease and renal failure approved by ACBS guidelines

Foods	Liver disease	Renal failure
Biscuits		
Aminex low-protein biscuits, cookies and rusks	✓	✓
Aproten biscuits		
dp low-protein butterscotch-flavoured or chocolate-flavoured chip cookies	✓	✓
Juvela low-protein cookies (chocolate chip, orange and cinnamon flavour)	✓	✓
Loprofin low-protein sweet biscuits, chocolate cream-filled biscuits, cookies (chocolate chip, cinnamon), wafers (orange, chocolate, vanilla)	✓	✓
Ultra PKU biscuits, cookies, savoy biscuits	✓	✓
Valpiform shortbread biscuits	✓	✓
Vita-Bite	✓	✓
Bread		
Juvela low-protein loaf (sliced and unsliced), bread rolls	✓	✓
Loprofin low-protein bread (sliced and unsliced), bread (canned, with or without salt), fibre bread (sliced and unsliced)	✓	✓
Ultra low-protein, canned white bread	✓	✓
Ultra PKU bread	✓	✓
Crispbread		
Aproten crispbread	✓	✓
Loprofin low-protein crackers	✓	✓
Egg replacer		
Ener G low-protein egg replacer	✓	✓
Loprofin egg replacer	✓	✓
Flour		
Ultra PKU flour	✓	✓
Mixes		
Aproten bread mix, cake mix	✓	✓
Juvela low-protein mix	✓	✓
Loprofin low-protein mix	✓	✓
Rite Diet low-protein baking mix, flour mix	✓	✓
Pizza bases		
Ultra PKU pizza base	✓	✓
Pasta		
Aproten annelini, ditalini, rigatini, spaghetti, tagliatelle	✓	✓

Table 8.11 Continued

Foods	Liver disease	Renal failure
Pasta		
Loprofin low-protein pasta (macaroni, penne, spaghetti long, pasta spirals, vermicelli)	✓	✓
Promin low-protein pasta (alphabets, macaroni, shells, shortcut spaghetti, spirals), pasta tricolour (alphabets, shells, spirals), pasta meal	✓	✓
Rice		
Aglutella low-protein rice	✓	✓
Promin pasta imitation rice	✓	✓
Supplements		
Alembicol D	✓	–
Generaid	✓	–
Generaid Plus	✓	–
Kindergen PROD	–	✓
Liquigen	✓	–
Medium Chain Triglyceride Oil	✓	–
Nepro	✓	✓
Renamil	–	✓
Sno-Pro Drink	–	✓
Suplena	✓	✓

✓ = recommended; – = items not recommended.

Useful addresses

The Coeliac Society
PO Box 220
High Wycombe
Bucks HP11 2HY
Tel: 01494 437278
www.coeliac.co.uk

National Society for Phenylketonuria (United Kingdom) Ltd
7 Lingey Lane
Wardley
Gateshead
Tyne & Wear NE10 8BR
Tel: 08456 039136
Helpline Tel: 0845 603 9136
web.ukonline.co.uk/nspku

Association for Glycogen Storage Disease (UK)
9 Lindop Road
Hale
Altrincham
Cheshire WA15 9DZ
Tel: 0161 980 7303
Helpline Tel: 0161 980 7303
www.agsd.org.uk

Organic Acidaemias UK (OAUK)
www.oauk.fsnet.co.uk

Maple Syrup Urine Disease Family Support
www.msud-support.org

British Kidney Patients Association
Oakhanger Place
Bordon
Hants GU35 9JZ
Tel: 01420 472021/2

National Kidney Federation
6 Stanley Street
Worksop
Nottinghamshire S81 7HX
Tel: 01909 487795
Helpline Tel: 0845 6010209
www.kidney.org.uk

British Liver Trust
Ransomes Europark
Ipswich IP3 9QG
Tel: 01473 276326
Helpline Tel: 0808 800 1000
www.britishlivertrust.org.uk

Children's Liver Disease Foundation
36 Great Charles Street
Birmingham B3 3JY
Tel: 0121 212 3839
www.childliverdisease.org

Cystic Fibrosis Trust
11 London Road
Bromley
Kent BR1 1BY
Tel: 020 8464 7211
www.cftrust.org.uk

The British Dietetic Association
5th Floor, Elizabeth House
22 Suffolk Street
Queensway
West Midlands B1 1LS
Tel: 0121 616 4900
www.bda.uk.com

9

Home parenteral nutrition

Pamela Mason

The administration of nutrients directly into the bloodstream is indicated when enteral feeding is not possible. Patients requiring such feeding are in a state of 'intestinal failure' and cannot be fed by mouth, by nasogastric feeding, or directly into the jejunum through a fine-tube jejunostomy. The common causes of intestinal failure are the presence of short bowel syndrome, intestinal fistula, peristaltic disorders, radiation enteritis and inflammatory bowel diseases (e.g. Crohn's disease).

Total parenteral nutrition has been widely used in hospitals since its introduction in the early 1960s. For some patients, however, the resumption of a normal life may only be possible through the introduction of intravenous feeding at home. It has also become more widely accepted that with adequate back-up provided by both family and healthcare professionals, and a high degree of individual motivation, patients usually recover more quickly in the familiar surroundings of their own home than when they are hospitalised for long periods.

The technique of home parenteral nutrition (HPN) was originally developed in the USA in the early 1970s, since when its use has become widespread throughout that country. In the UK, a few patients were initially treated with HPN in 1977 and 1978, but it was not until the start of the 1980s that the technique was introduced more widely. Even now, however, the number of new and long-term patients receiving treatment is low. It is currently estimated that there are about four or five HPN patients per million of the population (250–300 in total), and the number is fairly stable. In the immediate future, it is likely to remain rare for most pharmacists to encounter HPN patients outside the areas in which specialist centres are located (see below). Nevertheless, an awareness of the technique, and an understanding of the special problems that patients undergoing treatment with HPN may pose, may be required and are important aspects of the professional role of the pharmacist.

A register of HPN patients in the UK has been established at the Hope Hospital, Salford, and the majority of patients receiving treatment are currently managed by seven specialist centres (Hope Hospital, Salford; St Mark's Hospital, London; King's Cross Hospital, Dundee; St Mary's Hospital, Portsmouth; Royal Victoria Infirmary, Newcastle-upon-Tyne; Leeds General Infirmary; and the Northern General Hospital, Sheffield).

The benefits of HPN include improved patient survival, improved patient wellbeing, and cost savings. Home rather than hospital nutritional support is estimated to result in a saving of 50% for parenteral nutrition, i.e. about £150–175 per patient per day.

Indications for HPN

Severe gastrointestinal impairment may reduce the efficiency of absorption of food to such an extent that a patient cannot be nutritionally sustained on an oral diet alone. Most patients for whom HPN may be considered appropriate have already had unsuccessful oral dietary manipulations, been treated with antidiarrhoeal drugs, undergone extensive small-bowel resections, and frequently received nutritional supplements and possibly continuous enteral feeding. Despite all these measures, the patient remains malnourished, fluid and electrolyte levels remain abnormal, and long-term hospitalisation may be envisaged.

The most common indication for HPN is Crohn's disease, particularly after multiple small-bowel resections if the remaining portions of the bowel deteriorate. Other less frequent indications for HPN include radiation enteritis, thrombosis of the mesenteric artery or vein (which may produce gangrene of the small bowel and necessitate massive small bowel resections), enteric volvulus, intestinal scleroderma, pancreatitis and multiple enteric fistulae. HPN has also been introduced for the treatment of motility disorders, ulcerative colitis, pseudo-obstruction and, more controversially, malignancy of the intestine.

Without parenteral nutrition, the prognosis for many of these patients is poor. It must also be recognised that, in many cases, once parenteral nutrition has been initiated it may be a long-term requirement, although some patients have been selected for HPN as a temporary measure before surgical correction of the underlying disease. The age distribution of patients undergoing HPN reflects the incidence of the underlying conditions. Most patients are over 50 years of age, and this may have a bearing on the successful management of the treatment. Paediatric HPN has been initiated, but it demands significant motivation on the part of the child and their carers (usually the parents).

The technique of HPN administration

Routes of administration

Long-term intravenous catheterisation must be through a central rather than a peripheral vein. The administration of large volumes of solutions (even those that have been rendered isotonic) into a peripheral vein invariably results in thrombosis, caused by the irritant effects of the solution ingredients. To overcome this, the catheter is inserted through the chest wall into a wide-bore vessel, the cephalic vein, at the shoulder (Figure 9.1). The catheter crosses the subclavian vein and its tip lies in the superior vena cava just outside the right atrium. Alternative, but less commonly used, sites of catheterisation include the internal or external jugular vein, the femoral vein, and the muscular branches of the subclavian vein. The site of entry on the chest wall is chosen so that, when patients are sitting in a comfortable position, they can easily perform

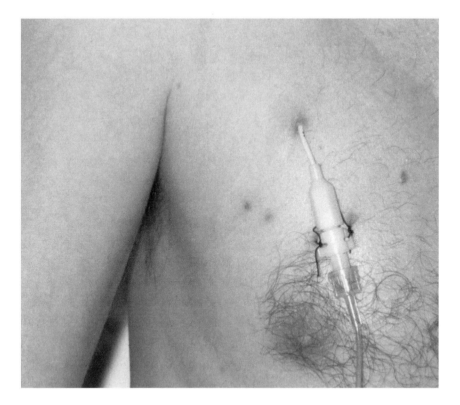

Figure 9.1 Entry point of catheter for parenteral nutrition. (Courtesy of Centre for Pharmacy Postgraduate Education.)

general catheter care themselves. Psychologically, it may also be important that the catheter entry site cannot be readily seen through outer
clothing. After each infusion the patency of the catheter is maintained
by a lock, which usually contains a solution of heparin. The catheter is
capped, allowing the patient to undertake normal activities. A subcutaneous port may be used in preference to a catheter, particularly for
patients who take part in swimming and other sporting activities.

A Dacron cuff placed around the catheter and situated under the
skin helps to keep the catheter in position. Fibrous tissue grows into the
cuff, holding it firmly in position in the subcutaneous tissues of the chest
wall and allowing it to remain in place, sometimes for many years. The
catheter is made of silicon rubber, which is inert when placed in living
tissue and does not corrode even after long-term use. It may have an
internal diameter of 1.0 mm (Broviac catheter) or 1.6 mm (Hickman
catheter). The use of the Hickman catheter may be preferable as it
becomes blocked less readily. The catheter is inserted aseptically in an
operating theatre, usually under local anaesthetic.

Equipment required

A variety of equipment is required for HPN, including:

- infusion devices
- HPN base solutions
- drug additives
- needles, syringes and alcohol wipes
- dressing-change kits
- intravenous sets, cassettes and filters
- intravenous pole
- catheter accessories.

A summary of the equipment requirements is presented below.

The catheter

The indwelling catheter is connected via an extension set to the control
centre for administration, the infusion pump (Figure 9.2). During the
period (usually through the day) that the patient is not connected to the
set, the extension tubing can be removed and the catheter irrigated with
heparinised saline. Antisepsis is maintained by capping off the catheter
and covering it with a sterile dressing, permitting the patient to go
to work or otherwise lead an active life. Strict adherence to aseptic

procedures by the patient during any catheter manipulations is essential to avoid infection complications (see Problems in HPN, below).

The pump

Fluids can be infused under gravity without the aid of a pump, but the degree of control over flow is poor and safety devices cannot be incorporated into the system. A greater degree of patient confidence and essential control over flow rates can be achieved with a volumetric infusion pump.

The pump is perhaps the most important part of the administration equipment. It can incorporate a range of alarms and sensors (e.g. to alert

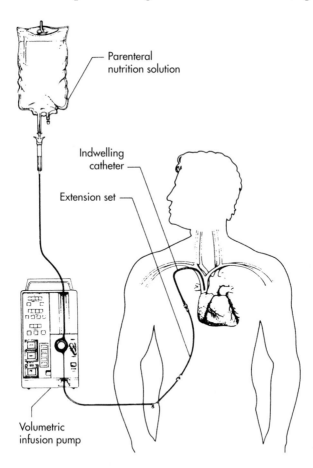

Parenteral
nutrition solution

Indwelling
catheter

Extension set

Volumetric
infusion pump

Figure 9.2 Home parenteral nutrition administration set. (Courtesy of Baxter Health-care.)

the patient and stop the infusion if air enters the system, or if the rate of flow changes). The patient is also made aware of the end of the infusion period. This is particularly important as most infusions are carried out overnight while the patient is asleep.

The infusion fluid

The administration of intravenous fluids in hospital was revolutionised and home therapy was made practicable only by the introduction in 1977 of disposable 3 L bags. These large-volume bags contain all the nutritional requirements of the patient and eliminate the need for multiple containers and connectors. All-in-one mixtures, compounded in the hospital pharmacy or a manufacturer's aseptic suite, can now be stored in a single container and delivered in cool-boxes direct to the patient's home. The patient must possess a refrigerator large enough to store up to two weeks' supply. (These refrigerators may on occasion be supplied by the fluids manufacturer.) Instability problems associated with some ingredients of the infusion fluid (e.g. vitamin supplements, see below) may require the patient to be trained to carry out aseptic additions to the bag at home. Where the patient is unable to carry out the aseptic manipulations satisfactorily, special local arrangements may be devised for additions to be made in an aseptic suite at a nearby hospital pharmacy.

Administration accessories

The range of peripherals required for satisfactory HPN is considerable. Gloves, towels and antiseptic solutions are required for catheter manipulations. Dressings, which are bulky and may require separate home storage facilities, must also be supplied. The patient, usually in association with the supplier, must ensure satisfactory stock control and rotation.

Solutions used in HPN

The solution used for HPN is essentially the same as that used in the hospital, being a combination of amino acids, dextrose, electrolytes, vitamins and minerals. An example of a typical adult HPN solution is given in Table 9.1. The bulk of most solutions is composed of energy sources, nitrogen and fluid. Other components may also be added in small volumes (e.g. vitamins, trace elements and minerals). The purpose of each of the ingredients is described briefly here.

Table 9.1 Total parenteral nutrition for adults

Components of a typical 3 L formula
Dextrose
Amino acids
Sodium chloride
Potassium chloride
Phosphate buffer
Mineral and trace element mixture
Water-soluble vitamin preparation
Antioxidant

Mineral and trace element mixtures include:
Calcium
Magnesium
Iron
Zinc
Manganese
Copper
Fluorine
Selenium
Chromium
Iodine

Water-soluble vitamin preparations, when reconstituted, contain:
Vitamin B_1
Vitamin B_2
Nicotinamide
Vitamin B_6
Pantothenic acid
Vitamin C
Biotin
Folic acid
Vitamin B_{12}

Insulin infusion
May be required if the patient is severely malnourished and glucose levels rise
above 10 mmol/L or glycosuria occurs

Preparations containing fat
Preparations containing fat, to which fat-soluble vitamins have been added, are
  commonly administered twice weekly through a peripheral infusion line.

Fat-soluble vitamin preparations contain:
Vitamin A
Vitamin D
Vitamin K_1

Adjustments are made to the above formulations based on the patient's particular requirements,
laboratory biochemical assay results and underlying condition.

Energy sources

Energy (calories) is provided by dextrose or fat emulsion, or both. Glucose is the carbohydrate of choice, as it is a normal constituent of blood. However, if large quantities (e.g. in excess of 300–400 g/day) are required, insulin must be given to increase the uptake of glucose into body tissues from the blood, encourage retention of nitrogen in muscle, and reduce the risks of rebound hypoglycaemia on cessation of administration.

Fructose, xylose and sorbitol have been used as alternatives to glucose, but with limited efficacy.

Energy requirements may also be supplied by fat preparations, which are commonly administered as lipid emulsions, although the emulsion cannot be mixed in the same container as synthetic crystalline amino acids. One advantage of the use of a fat emulsion is that it is isotonic with blood, unlike the hypertonic high-concentration glucose solution. Most lipid solutions, which are essential as a vehicle for the administration of fat-soluble vitamins and for the prevention of fatty-acid deficiencies, are given in two 500 mL infusions each week in place of the standard nutritional solution.

Nitrogen source

Nitrogen is required to maintain the 'nitrogen balance' in the body, which can be measured by calculating the nitrogen intake and assessing the nitrogen content of blood, urea, and body fluid lost. Most patients selected for parenteral nutrition are in a state of negative nitrogen balance (i.e. their protein and amino acid stores are depleted), and the aim of many forms of parenteral nutrition is to achieve a positive nitrogen balance. The nitrogen balance cannot be considered in isolation, however, as energy sources (see above) must be given at the same time so that the amino acids can be used as muscle-building components, not as catabolic agents.

L-Amino acids are used as the source of protein in the intravenous diet. The amount of protein administered can vary from 9 to 14 g nitrogen (1 g of nitrogen is equivalent to 6.25 g of protein). The exact amount required is assessed during hospitalisation.

Amino acids are classed as essential or non-essential. The eight essential amino acids (valine, leucine, isoleucine, threonine, methionine, phenylalanine, tryptophan and lysine) cannot be synthesised in the human body and must therefore be supplied in the diet. However, it is usual to include both essential and non-essential amino acids in the nutritional package, as the synthesis of non-essential amino acids may be impaired in patients who are ill. It is likely that some non-essential amino acids are in fact essential during illness, and the value of supplementing HPN solutions with, for example, additional glutamine, carnitine and extra branched-chain amino acids, continues to be debated.

Trace elements

As their name implies, only very small quantities of the elements are required in the diet, but their absence may produce a significant deterioration in body functioning. It is thought unlikely that a patient undergoing short-term parenteral nutrition will develop such deficiencies. However, long-term administration requires the addition of these elements to the parenteral solution.

Copper is necessary for the normal maturation of red blood cells and for the production of certain enzymes. In its absence, neutropenia and anaemia may occur. Zinc and manganese are common prerequisites for the functioning of many enzyme systems. A deficiency of zinc has been reported to produce skin and mucous membrane lesions, dermatitis, diarrhoea, depression and hair loss. Chromium deficiency is recognised in long-term (more than three years) parenteral therapy, resulting in glucose intolerance and neuropathy. A lack of selenium may produce muscle pain and tenderness, and cardiomyopathy. Deficiencies of iodine, cobalt, and iron have also been reported.

Electrolytes and minerals

Many patients who require parenteral nutrition may have disturbed electrolyte levels (e.g. metabolic acidosis). Equally, the initial requirements for electrolytes can vary, depending on whether large amounts of fluids or water have been lost. While the patient is in hospital, plasma electrolyte levels are measured and renal function is assessed to determine current electrolyte levels. Subsequently, blood sodium and potassium levels can be monitored daily, and weekly checks can be made on phosphate, magnesium and calcium levels.

Sodium is the predominant extracellular cation and plays an important role in the maintenance of blood volume. About 100–120 mmol sodium are required each day by a patient whose fluid balance is stable.

Potassium is the major intracellular cation and is important in cardiac function. As potassium cannot be conserved by the body, its plasma level is dependent on renal function. The average daily requirement of potassium is about 70 mmol, but may be considerably higher if a large amount of fluid is lost (e.g. in vomiting and diarrhoea).

Calcium, phosphate and magnesium levels also require regular monitoring. Loss of magnesium may be high in patients with severe diarrhoea or vomiting. Severely malnourished patients may need more phosphate than normal, to prevent the development of muscle weakness and impaired white cell function.

Vitamins

One of the main problems in providing a total nutritional package for the home patient is caused by the relative instability of vitamins in the solutions administered. The degradation of vitamins is encouraged by exposure to ultraviolet light and to warm temperatures. Vitamin A may be adsorbed to the container material, although this problem has been reduced with the introduction of new container materials (see below). To overcome this problem, all water- and fat-soluble vitamins (except vitamin K) can be given separately as a once-weekly intramuscular injection, or even as an oral supplement if the patient is capable of absorbing it. Alternatively, the patient can be trained in the aseptic addition of a mixed vitamin preparation to the infusion solution.

Folic acid is required for the maturation of red and white blood cells, and folic acid deficiency is common in infusion feeding. This is overcome by including it in multiple vitamin preparations.

Labelling and storage

Solutions for HPN are supplied in 'all-in-one' 3 L bags made of a non-plasticised material, ethylenevinylacetate (EVA). The containers are labelled with the patient's name, the total container constituents, the expiry date, storage conditions, and specific infusion instructions. The container is encased in a foil sleeve, which protects the fluid from the light. It is refrigerated before dispatch and is transported to the patient in a cool-box. Each cool-box can carry up to five 3 L containers.

If the bags are correctly stored in a refrigerator, they have a shelf-life of up to two weeks. However, once additions (e.g. of vitamins) have been made, an expiry date of four days is commonly recommended. Once the container has been removed from the refrigerator, it must be used within 24 hours.

Rate of administration

The infusion rate and time of administration are selected to cause minimal disruption to the patient's lifestyle. Most 3 L solutions can be infused at a constant rate over an 8–14-hour period. The infusion rate at the end of this period can be gradually reduced to prevent the development of hypoglycaemia, caused by the high levels of circulating insulin. Replacing the 3 L nutritional package with a 500 mL fat emulsion (see above) can reduce the infusion period to four hours.

Fluids can be given at night while patients are in bed to allow them to follow a normal daytime routine.

Training the patient before hospital discharge

Any patients who are given responsibility for managing their condition outside the 'protected' environment of the hospital must be suitably trained in the techniques they are required to perform. This will enable them to gain confidence in their therapy and to recognise when problems have occurred. Equally important for patients is the identification of an individual within the hospital to whom they can turn if problems arise. Although the length of time spent on training can vary, up to a week may be required for the patient to learn how to care for the catheter and its entry site and how to heparinise the catheter port each day. A further two weeks may be needed for acquiring skills in making aseptic additions to the 3 L bags (when required), in using the infusion pump and recording daily weight and urine output, and in making temporary repairs to the catheter.

Patients are usually trained in the hospital by a specialist nurse, with input from other members of the nutritional team, including the pharmacist. A nutritional unit may furnish an area or room in the hospital so that it resembles a typical room that might be used in the patient's home to carry out the manipulations.

The importance of aseptic technique in catheter manipulation is paramount, and patients invariably need a detailed explanation of the reasons for this. They also need to have demonstrated their skill in aseptic manipulations (e.g. changing the catheter dressing) on several occasions before they are discharged. They must demonstrate their competence in attaching the infusion bag to the infusion line; running through the solution and connecting it to the indwelling catheter; and, after completion of the infusion, flushing the catheter port with heparinised saline, capping it, and applying a sterile dressing.

In all aspects of patient training the support of another member of the family is usually considered essential. Ideally, both the patient and his or her partner are trained in all techniques. The amount and complexity of the information they are required to assimilate may appear daunting, and all verbal and practical advice is reinforced by written information that can be read and referred to after discharge.

The patient is taught to monitor weight and urine output each day. In conjunction with blood electrolyte, creatinine, urea and nitrogen monitoring, these measures provide an accurate assessment of the patient's fluid balance. The patient is advised of the degree of variation that can be tolerated and those that require referral to the nutritional team.

Satisfactory training does not require a patient to be of above-average intelligence: what is essential is the ability to carry out instructions in a logical and sensible fashion. One of the greatest incentives to the successful adoption of the HPN programme is patients' awareness that their general health improves significantly after parenteral feeding begins.

Problems in HPN

Complications of HPN may be due to problems related to mechanical disturbances in the blood vessels and the catheter, an imbalance in the nutritional programme, or the presence of infection. Patients may also experience psychological problems relating to the use of parenteral nutrition. Pharmacists should be aware of the interrelationships between each of these potential problem areas and the effects they may have on the successful management and quality of life of the patient.

All of these problems can also arise in the hospital environment. The major difference, however, is that the patient at home is not under constant specialised supervision and may delay asking for help. It is therefore important that both patients and pharmacists are aware of the outward signs of the development of problems (see Table 9.2). On the positive side, there is a significantly reduced likelihood of bacterial challenge in the home. Also, many patients are highly motivated in the management of their condition, thus reducing the likelihood that major problems will occur.

Mechanical problems

The introduction of a catheter into the chest wall is a potential source of damage to the vessels and lung membranes through which it is passed.

Table 9.2 Signs indicating catheter complications

Complication	Signs and symptoms
Infection	
Systemic	Lethargy, fever, sweating and chills
Exit site	Localised tenderness, redness and swelling
Thrombosis	Veins in the shoulder and anterior chest wall distended; arm and facial swelling; pain in the shoulder, neck or throat, lachrymation and rhinorrhoea
Air embolism	Chest pain, shortness of breath, cough
Breakage of catheter	Leakage of blood or parenteral fluid
Dislodgement of catheter	Chest swelling; pain in the neck and shoulder regions

Pneumothorax and fatal air embolisms are unlikely to arise once the patient has been stabilised in hospital, but the daily handling of the catheter generates some risk of breakage and of the introduction of air into the system.

External catheter problems commonly arise through wear and tear of the hub of the catheter, generated by repeated connection to and disconnection from the giving set. The hub may become cracked, causing fluid to leak. Repair kits are available which preclude the need for complete catheter replacement.

Internal blockage of the catheter is a serious problem. This is commonly caused by thrombosis, possibly as a consequence of inadequate flushing of the catheter port with heparinised saline. If the blockage develops in an interval between HPN administration and is noticed by the patient within an hour, it may be possible to dissolve it with an injection of urokinase before the catheter becomes irretrievably damaged. However, longer-term blockages may be impossible to clear, and these require replacement of the catheter. Blockage of the catheter during HPN administration will reduce the flow rate and increase back-pressure to the pump, which may activate an alarm system.

Blockage of the subclavian vein or the superior vena cava requires urgent hospitalisation for removal of the catheter. The outward signs of blood vessel blockage include swelling of the neck and head on the same side of the body as the catheter, and difficulty in rotating the head. Similar signs may also be produced by intravascular and extravascular displacement of the catheter.

Metabolic complications

The development of metabolic complications can be prevented by careful monitoring by the patient, which in turn emphasises the importance of adequate training before discharge (see above). Most metabolic complications are rare once the patient has been stabilised on a particular treatment regimen, but liver complications remain a long-term possible complication for HPN patients.

Water and electrolyte imbalances may occur, causing overhydration or dehydration and hypo- or hypernatraemia. Changes in osmolality may accompany changes in sodium ion and blood glucose concentrations. Imbalances may arise in levels of potassium, calcium, magnesium, phosphate and vitamins. The maximum period of infusion is limited to 10–12 hours daily by the development of the acute glucose intolerance syndrome, which produces sleep disturbances, anxiety, nausea and vomiting, abdominal cramps and sweating.

The likelihood that a deficiency in essential fatty acids will occur is minimised by administering some of the calorific requirements as an intravenous fat emulsion (see above). Trace element supplements are also necessary to prevent deficiencies. Metabolic bone diseases have been reported in a number of patients undergoing long-term parenteral therapy. This may be caused by a form of vitamin D toxicity and is characterised by hypercalciuria, periodic hypercalcaemia and osteomalacia. The patient may complain of bone pain and be particularly susceptible to fractures of the ribs and pelvis. Increased calcium supplementation combined with a reduction in the vitamin D content of the parenteral fluid may eliminate this problem.

Infections

Catheter-related sepsis and infections of the channel through the subcutaneous tissue may be consequences of poor management of the entry site of the catheter. Infection of the exit site may be shown by the presence of pain, redness and tenderness around the injection site, commonly caused by staphylococci. Infection which has spread to the subcutaneous tunnel leading to the Dacron cuff is commonly due to staphylococci or candida. If infectious symptoms occur, the catheter should not be used and the patient should be urgently referred to the hospital. A positive culture report may require removal of the catheter and treatment with an appropriate antimicrobial for five to seven days.

Prophylactic antimicrobial therapy may be necessary in the event of unrelated minor surgical or investigative procedures (e.g. dental extraction, dilatation and curettage, or colonoscopy). Patients should be advised to consult their general practitioner or hospital nutritional unit for further information.

Psychological and social problems

The ability of the patient to adapt to parenteral nutrition may depend on the degree of planning and counselling possible before HPN is begun. A patient who has been severely ill for a long time with Crohn's disease is more likely to respond positively to HPN than a previously independent patient who has undergone unexpected trauma and for whom HPN is the only way in which a normal home life may be resumed. In both instances, patients must adjust to altered patterns of body functions and eating. They must accept that they have to rely on the supply of nutrition from the hospital or from a distribution company. Some patients may feel trapped by their dependence.

The signs that readjustment is difficult or that patients are rebelling against their treatment can vary. Clinical depression occurs in up to 20% of patients, and may alternate with nausea, sleep disturbances and significant fluctuations in mood. Staff involved in the management of HPN patients must be alert to these signs and be aware that they may also accompany metabolic disturbances.

The ability to readjust may be hampered by night-time administration of the nutritional fluid. Disruption to sleep patterns, increased frequency of micturition, and polyuria caused by the administration of large volumes of fluid can aggravate depressive tendencies when treatment is initiated. Many patients, however, find that, if early problems are explained and accepted and the positive benefits of their treatment are emphasised, they can quickly learn to adapt.

Patients also have to come to terms with the loss of 'social' eating. Some may react particularly severely to the loss of the pleasure of tasting foods; to overcome this they may sample and subsequently eject a bolus of food.

The quality of life of a patient may be measured by the resumption of normal daily activities and the degree of dependence on others. It has been estimated that most adult patients can resume full- or part-time work or fulfil their domestic responsibilities in the same manner as before therapy began. This is particularly true of patients with Crohn's disease, which possibly reflects the general improvement in health such patients may experience when enteral feeding is stopped. A smaller proportion may not feel confident enough about managing their condition to resume work, but may be able to carry out most of the necessary manipulations for themselves in the home. A minority may require major assistance in the management of their condition, although it is expected that this proportion could decrease further with improved patient selection.

Drug administration

Many patients on HPN are unable to take drugs orally because they are unable to absorb them effectively. This means that another route of administration must be used. Any parenteral medication required is best given into a peripheral vein well away from the entry site of the catheter delivering the feed. However, if the patient has poor venous access this may not be possible, and a double-lumen catheter may be used, with one lumen dedicated to the administration of nutrients and the other used for other purposes (e.g. medication administration).

Drugs should not normally be added directly to parenteral feeds because of the potential for stability and incompatibility problems. Some drugs may interact not only with the parenteral nutrition solution but also with the container and/or giving set. Less is known about inter-actions between drugs and parenteral solutions than between drugs and enteral feeds. However, specific examples include a reduction in the effect of warfarin in the presence of lipid emulsions, and a fall in theo-phylline levels when the amino acid concentration of the feed is increased. Serum phenytoin levels may fall when parenteral nutrition is given, interfering with seizure control, but evidence for this is limited to single case reports.

Useful addresses

British Association of Parenteral and Enteral Nutrition (BAPEN)
PO Box 922
Maidenhead
Berkshire SL6 4SH
www.bapen.org.uk

British Pharmaceutical Nutrition Group
www.bpng.co.uk

Patients on Intravenous and Nasogastric Nutrition Therapy (PINNT)
PO Box 3126
Christchurch
Dorset BH23 2XS
Tel: 01202 481625
www.pinnt.com

10

Home enteral nutrition

Pamela Mason

Enteral nutrition is usually taken to mean nutrition support provided in the form of nutritional supplements (e.g. sip feeds) or a feed delivered by tube into the patient's gastrointestinal tract. This type of nutritional support is required in patients who are nutritionally 'at risk' but who have a functioning gut. If the gut is not functioning parenteral nutrition is needed, which can also be given at home (see Chapter 9).

Since the early 1990s there has been a rapid increase in the number of patients receiving enteral nutrition at home. By 2001, it was estimated that there were nearly 16 000 such patients in Britain. In 1997, home enteral nutrition (HEN) had become more common in the community than in the hospital environment. Factors which have contributed to this include the general shift in treatment towards primary care, advances in technology, changes in clinical practice, and an awareness among clinicians that services exist in the community to support patients at home.

Pharmacists have traditionally been the main sources of supply of enteral feeds in the community, although some home care companies are now fulfilling this role to some extent. However, pharmacists can still have a significant input into the care of patients on enteral feeds, whether supplying the products or not. Many patients on enteral feeds are also on medication, and pharmacists can advise on the choice and administration of drugs in tube-fed patients. In addition, pharmacists can help to ensure patient compliance with both medication and feeds, as well as advising on problems the patient or carer may have with the administration of the feed or use of the feeding equipment.

Enteral feeds are indicated in a variety of conditions (see below), but the issue of fundamental importance is that the patient is at risk of becoming, or may have become, malnourished.

Malnutrition

Incidence

Malnutrition is an important public health problem in the UK and is not, as is often thought, a condition restricted to developing countries. In England, 6.9% of women and 4.2% of men are underweight; in Scotland the figures are 8.7% for women and 5.1% for men. This translates to a total of about 3.2 million people in England, Wales and Scotland who are underweight. Older people are especially at risk, with between 3 and 6% of community-based and up to 16% of institutionalised elderly patients considered to be at risk of or suffering from malnutrition. This means that of the 150 000 people over the age of 75 years in long-term care, 24 000 could be malnourished. In addition, up to 40% of adults and 60% of older people are malnourished on admission to hospital. To put the problem in context, in the average parliamentary constituency of 90 000 people, up to 5000 are at risk of malnutrition, and this includes 980 people over the age of 65.

Causes of malnutrition

Undernutrition has many causes that are related to physical and psychosocial problems and public health issues (e.g. poverty, education, and the general health of the nation). It may develop as a result of reduced dietary intake, increased nutritional requirements, or an inability to absorb or utilise certain nutrients. Almost any chronic disease can lead to anorexia, tissue catabolism, and/or increased requirement for nutrients. Conditions such as arthritis or muscle weakness can result in problems with shopping, preparing food and eating; gastrointestinal disease (e.g. Crohn's disease, coeliac disease, and nausea and vomiting) can lead to anorexia and malabsorption. Multiple drug use, usually an indicator of chronic disease, should not be forgotten as a potential cause of undernutrition, particularly in someone who is already vulnerable because of a poor diet. Several drugs can cause confusion, sedation and gastrointestinal side-effects, all of which can lead to poor dietary intake and problems with absorption.

Consequences and costs of malnutrition

Undernutrition can become manifest in several ways, but the most obvious consequences are weight loss, progressive muscle wasting and lethargy. Malnourished people often have an impaired immune response, resulting in a predisposition to infection and poor wound healing. Recovery from illness may be delayed and the length of hospital stays increased.

The health, social and economic costs of undernutrition are not accurately known but are likely to be substantial, with the main burden lying in the community. Studies indicate that patients with gastro-intestinal, respiratory and neurological disease-related malnutrition have a 6% higher GP consultation rate, are given 9% more prescriptions and have a 26% higher hospital admission rate than those who are well nourished, costing an estimated £7.3 million per 100 000 patients to the NHS.

Indications for enteral nutrition

When adequate nutrition cannot be achieved via the oral route artificial nutritional support may be indicated and, provided the patient can digest and absorb nutrients adequately, enteral feeding is suitable. It is only when the patient cannot absorb nutrients (i.e. when the gut is not functioning) that parenteral nutrition is necessary. The enteral route should be chosen wherever possible because it has a reduced risk of complications. It is also cheaper and easier to manage and helps to pre-serve gut mucosal integrity. However, the patient must be at the centre of any decision taken about nutritional support, and health professionals have a responsibility to take the patient's wishes into account and respect them.

Conditions in which enteral feeding may be indicated include:

- major surgery, particularly to the face, head, or neck
- injury to the head or neck
- head and neck cancer
- neurological conditions (e.g. cerebral vascular accident, multiple sclerosis, Parkinson's disease and motor neurone disease)
- gastrointestinal disease (e.g. inflammatory bowel disease, oeso-phageal obstruction and short bowel syndrome)
- cystic fibrosis
- anorexia nervosa
- burns and sepsis
- HIV/AIDS
- organ system failure (e.g. renal, hepatic, cardiac or respiratory).

The technique of HEN

Routes of administration

Enteral feeds can be given by various routes (Figure 10.1).

Nasogastric (NG)

This involves tube feeding via the nose into the stomach. It is the most common type of enteral feeding but should only be used short term (i.e.

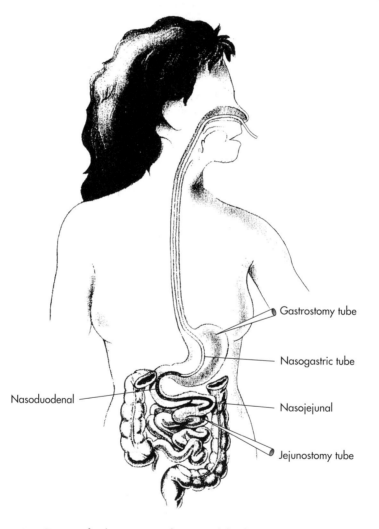

Gastrostomy tube

Nasogastric tube

Nasoduodenal

Nasojejunal

Jejunostomy tube

Figure 10.1 Routes of administration for enteral feeds.

for up to two weeks). Contraindications to NG feeding include gastro-oesophageal reflux, upper gastrointestinal bleeding and inadequate gastric emptying. NG tubes have a fine bore and are generally made of PVC, silk or polyurethane. Wide-bore tubes, often used in the past, are no longer recommended because they are uncomfortable. They can also lead to impaired cardiac sphincter function, increasing the risk of gastro-oesophageal reflux and aspiration, and the gastric juices can make the tubes stiffen. There is a risk of gastric aspiration with NG feeding, and the tube must be carefully sited. Some tubes have a weighted end, which makes use of gravity to help with their placement.

Nasoduodenal

This involves placing the tube beyond the stomach in the duodenum, which is a useful route when there are problems with gastric emptying. The risk of aspiration is reduced, but it may be difficult to prevent movement of the tip of the tube back into the stomach. This route is appropriate only in acute hospitals (e.g. in intensive care units) and is not used for home enteral feeding.

Nasojejunal

This involves passing the feeding tube into the jejunum. The risk of aspiration is minimised but, like nasoduodenal feeding, it is suitable only in an acute setting and not at home.

Percutaneous endoscopic gastrostomy (PEG)

This involves passing a tube endoscopically into the stomach through the abdominal wall. It is used for long-term feeding and is therefore common in patients on HEN. Indications include stroke when the patient has failed to regain the swallowing reflex after several weeks, multiple sclerosis, cystic fibrosis in patients who require long-term supplementation, and injury to or cancer of the head or neck. PEG tubes are made of polyurethane and are designed for long-term use of from one to five years. This is a useful method for patients who tend to remove NG tubes, as PEG tubes are less visible and far more discreet. However, it is not suitable for patients with morbid obesity, previous gastric surgery, gastric varices, massive ascites, peritoneal dialysis, Crohn's disease and hepatomegaly.

Button gastrostomy

This involves the use of a tube inserted into an existing gastrostomy tract when the original PEG tube needs to be replaced. A button gastrostomy tube is held in place by a balloon on the inside of the stomach wall, and the button lies completely flat against the patient's abdomen. These tubes are useful in patients needing long-term gastrostomy access, particularly those who dislike the appearance of a PEG tube, but there is a risk of leakage round the site of insertion.

Percutaneous endoscopic jejunostomy (PEJ)

This is a tube placed endoscopically through the PEG tract into the stomach, past the pylorus and into the jejunum. It is essentially an extension of a PEG. The risk of feed aspiration is minimal, but this type of tube is used in a limited number of patients who require postpyloric feeding.

Surgical jejunostomy

This is a tube placed directly into the jejunum through the abdominal wall. The procedure is carried out under general anaesthetic, and is used when gastrointestinal feeding is indicated but the stomach is not viable and an endoscopy is not feasible.

Equipment

An enteral feeding system usually consists of three parts: a pump, a reservoir and a giving set (Figures 10.2 and 10.3).

The pump

The pump is used to deliver the feed at a constant rate. It consists of a rate control device, a locking device to hold the giving set in place, a drive arm, an alarm to indicate if the tube is blocked or the reservoir empty, a clip or clamp to secure it to a pole, and a mains power connection. Some pumps also have a rechargeable battery.

The flow rate is set to suit the patient and the feed regimen and can be varied. Once set, the pump does not need frequent attention to adjust the flow rate. An enteral feed pump must be used; pumps designed for parenteral nutrition generate higher pressures and are unsuitable.

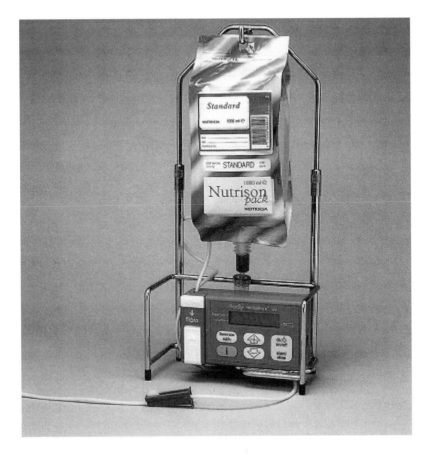

Figure 10.2 Mini-drip stand showing an enteral feed connected to a pump. (Courtesy of Nutricia Clinical Care.)

The reservoir

Most tube feeds are provided in 500 mL bottles or packs which can take a nasogastric giving set directly, thus minimising the risk of contamination. Products that have to be reconstituted or diluted and poured into another reservoir are not recommended for HEN unless there is no suitable ready-to-use feed. There is usually a means of securing the reservoir so that it can be hung on a pole, birdcage stand or curtain rail for administration.

The giving set

The giving set usually consists of three parts, and all manufacturers produce a giving set compatible with their own bottles. The viewing

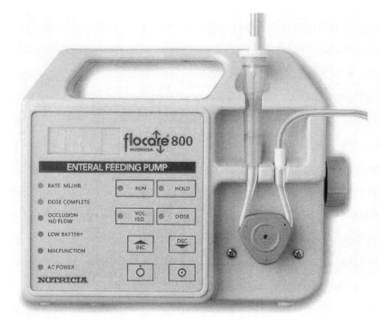

Figure 10.3 An enteral feeding pump. (Courtesy of Nutricia Clinical Care.)

chamber is designed to allow the flow rate to be checked. It is situated just below the reservoir and must be primed when the feed is set up, so that it is partly filled with liquid; this makes it easier to see what is happening. A clamp is used to occlude the tubing when the reservoir is first connected; it is also used to control the flow rate when a pump is not used. When a pump is used, the clamp must be fully open. A naso-gastric tube attachment is designed to connect to the feeding tube (nasogastric or gastrostomy). Some giving sets have a port for giving drugs.

Types of feed

A wide range of feeds is available. Like a normal diet they contain protein, fat, carbohydrate, water, vitamins and minerals. Some contain dietary fibre; others contain one or more of a growing range of novel substrates thought to be beneficial for certain patients. Most feeds are nutritionally complete and can be used as the sole source of nutrition. Most are gluten free and many are also lactose free. The choice of feed is governed by the patient's nutritional status. This will depend on a number of factors, including disease state, which may modify the amounts and proportions of nutrients required, and the level of tissue catabolism. Nutrient requirements are calculated and the route of administration chosen, but other factors should also be considered (e.g. flavours, feed viscosity, osmolality, and compatibility of the preparation with the feeding equipment).

Enteral feeds can be divided into several categories.

Standard feeds

Often described as polymeric, these feeds provide 1 kcal/mL and contain whole protein, fat (from vegetable oils), glucose polymers (usually maltodextrin), vitamins and minerals. They are suitable for patients with normal nutritional requirements and a functioning gastrointestinal tract.

High-energy feeds

These are similar to standard feeds in composition except that their energy content is higher (1.3–2 kcal/mL). They are indicated for patients with high energy requirements or for those with normal energy requirements who are fluid restricted.

Elemental feeds

These contain nutrients in their most easily absorbable form (i.e. protein in the form of amino acids, fat mainly as medium-chain triglycerides (MCTs), and carbohydrate in the form of mono- and disaccharides). They are indicated for patients with severe malabsorption problems (e.g. Crohn's disease, bowel fistulae, short bowel syndrome) or for those who are transferring to enteral feeding after a period on parenteral nutrition. Energy content varies between 1 and 1.3 kcal/mL. Elemental feeds are more expensive than standard feeds. They used to be more unpalatable, but the taste has improved considerably in recent years.

Semi-elemental feeds

As the name suggests, these are similar to elemental feeds but the protein is provided as a mixture of peptides and amino acids rather than just amino acids.

Fibre-containing feeds

These are similar to standard feeds but contain dietary fibre. They are indicated for patients on long-term enteral feeding to help maintain healthy bowel function. The fibre acts as a substrate for the colonic microflora and produces long-chain fatty acids. These promote the absorption of water and sodium, and fibre-containing feeds may therefore have a role in the management of diarrhoea, which is often a problem in tube-fed patients.

Paediatric feeds

Feeds which are nutritionally complete for adults are not necessarily suitable for children between one and six years of age, and specially formulated enteral feeds are available for children.

Feeds containing novel substances

There has been a great deal of research in recent years showing the potential benefits of a range of substances. These include glutamine, arginine, nucleotides (i.e. precursors of RNA and DNA), omega-3 fatty acids and antioxidants. Suggested benefits include improved immune function, preservation of gut mucosal integrity, and increased resistance to infection.

Disease-specific feeds

Some feeds are designed to take account of the needs of patients with specific diseases (e.g. hepatic and renal failure). Such feeds are high in energy to minimise urine output, but low in protein to avoid exacerbation of uraemia. They contain reduced levels of sodium, potassium, phosphate and other electrolytes.

For examples of common feeds prescribable under the Advisory Committee on Borderline Substances guidelines, see Table 10.1. Details of dietary products prescribable for special disease states (e.g. renal and hepatic impairment, inborn errors of metabolism and coeliac disease) can be found in Chapter 8.

Administration schedules

Enteral feeds may be administered by continuous or intermittent infusion or as a bolus. Continuous infusion may be appropriate for patients

Table 10.1 Common examples of enteral feeds suitable for tube feeding approved by Advisory Committee on Borderline Substances (ACBS) guidelines

Standard feeds
Ensure
Fresubin Liquid
Isosource Standard
Novasource GI control
Nutrison Soya
Nutrison Standard
Nutrison MCT
Osmolite
Peptisorb
Sondalis ISO

High-energy feeds
Enrich Plus
Ensure Plus
Fresubin 750 MCT
Fresubin 1000 Complete
Isosource Energy
Nutrison Energy
Osmolite Plus
Peptisorb
Sondalis 1.5

Elemental and semi-elemental feeds
Elemental 028
Emsogen
Nutrison Pepti
Pepdite
Peptamen
Perative
Survimed OPD

Fibre-containing feeds
Enrich
Fresubin Energy Fibre
Fresubin 1000 and 1200 Complete
Fresubin Isofibre
Isosource Fibre
Jevity
Jevity Plus
Novasource GI Control
Nutrison Multi Fibre
Sondalis Fibre

Paediatric feeds (for children 1–6 years)
Frebini
Infatrini (for infants 0–12 months)

Table 10.1 Continued

Paediatric feeds (for children 1–6 years)
Nutrini Extra
Nutrini Fibre
Nutrini Standard
Paediasure Liquid
Paediasure Liquid with Fibre
Paediasure Plus
Sondalis Junior

---

unable to tolerate large volumes of feed (e.g. patients with partial or total gastrectomy), but this method does not allow for daily activities without being attached to the pump. Intermittent infusion, with breaks of six hours or more, should be started as soon as possible to suit the patient's needs. Bolus feeding involves inputting a volume of feed through the tube at regular intervals, mimicking meal and snack times. This type of feeding should only be given when the patient is being fed into the stomach, not the jejunum, because the jejunum, having a smaller volume than the stomach, is unable to cope with large quantities of liquid.

Problems with HEN

Enteral nutrition is a safer technique than parenteral nutrition, but it can nevertheless be associated with problems. A knowledge of these problems and their resolution is important for pharmacists involved in the care of these patients.

Gastrointestinal symptoms represent the main type of problem experienced by patients on enteral nutrition, both in hospital and at home. There can also be problems with the equipment, including the pump and the feeding tube; for patients with a gastrostomy, there may also be problems with the stoma.

Gastrointestinal symptoms

Diarrhoea is one of the most common problems in tube-fed patients, with an incidence of 10–25%. There are several possible causes: contamination of the feed or the equipment is a prime cause, and it is vital that patients understand the importance of good hygienic practice and maintaining it (see Table 10.2). Enteral feeds are excellent growth media and can become heavily contaminated if these basic rules are not

Table 10.2 Good microbiological practice for enteral feeding

- Hands should be washed thoroughly before handling feeds and feed equipment
- Feeds, feed reservoirs and giving sets should be discarded every 24 hours
- All equipment should be kept sealed in its packaging until required for use, and thereafter handled minimally
- Once opened, feeds should be refrigerated and used within 24 hours. However, they should be allowed to come to room temperature before use
- Decanting feeds into separate containers should be avoided as this increases the risk of contamination. Any feed that has been decanted should normally be discarded after four hours
- Enteral feeding tubes should be flushed with 30 mL of water before and after feeding and before and after drug administration. A 50 mL syringe should be used for this purpose and tap water is suitable unless the patient is being fed jejunally, when sterile water should be used

---

followed. When patients become used to their feeding regimen they may become less careful, and pharmacists can reinforce the importance of good practice.

Diarrhoea can also be caused by over-rapid infusion of the feed and a feed that is too cold. Feeds should always be allowed to reach room temperature if they have been stored in the refrigerator. The patient's condition can also lead to diarrhoea. Any condition of malabsorption (e.g. inflammatory bowel disorders, short bowel syndrome and intestinal mucosal atrophy) can cause diarrhoea, for which feeding with a semi-elemental or elemental formula may be better. Medication (e.g. antibiotics, antacids and laxatives) is a common cause of diarrhoea in tube-fed patients, and pharmacists should be aware of the need to conduct regular medication reviews in these patients.

Constipation may also occur, possibly caused by medication, insufficient fluid or inadequate fibre intake. Several feeds contain dietary fibre (see Table 10.1), and these may be better to use. Other gastrointestinal problems include nausea and vomiting and abdominal distension, possibly caused by delayed gastric emptying and requiring the choice of feeding route or the feed to be reconsidered. In addition, nausea and vomiting may occur as a result of an over-rapid infusion rate or feed contamination. The flavour of the feed may also have an effect: some flavours may make a patient feel sick.

Tube-fed patients may experience a sore mouth, which can be remedied by good oral hygiene, or by the use of a mouthwash, spray or anaesthetic gel. If the mouth is particularly dry an artificial saliva spray can be applied.

Problems with the equipment

Problems can occur with the pump or the feeding tube. Most pumps are supplied by a central equipment store run by the local hospital or by the company that supplies the feed. All companies offer prompt servicing and maintenance services.

Tube blockage is a common problem, to which the patient will be alerted by the occlusion alarm on the pump. If the patient is following the provided protocol and flushing the tube regularly, it should not block. Very occasionally, however, tubes can block because they become embedded in the stomach tissue (which requires hospital treatment) or kinked. Drugs, particularly if administered inappropriately (see below), may also block the tube.

A blockage can be relieved by water. Other substances have also been used (e.g. carbonated water, pineapple juice, cranberry juice, water containing lemon juice, or bicarbonate solution) and the patient should have been given advice on this by the hospital. Occasionally, pancreatic enzyme solution may be injected into the tube and left for several hours. However, there is no substantial evidence for the value of any substance other than water.

Tubes may split and/or crack, and if so the district nurse or the community dietitian should be alerted. Poor NG or NJ tube positioning, or constant displacement of the tube, can lead to reflux of the feed and/or gastrointestinal contents. This can often be improved by keeping the patient's head elevated at 30° while feeding and for one hour afterwards.

Problems with the stoma

Like any other stoma, a gastrostomy or jejunostomy may cause problems (e.g. the surrounding skin may become red and irritated). This can be due to gastric leakage, a discharging stoma or an allergic reaction. Management is best achieved by keeping the skin clean and dry and applying a barrier cream and/or waterproof plaster. In the case of suspected allergy an alternative soap or cream may be tried, and if the stoma shows signs of infection (e.g. discharge of pus, foul-smelling brown fluid) antibiotics may be required. However, regular cleaning of the stoma can help to reduce the need for antibiotics.

Psychological and social problems

Most people take for granted the ability to eat and drink normally, and enteral feeding can lead to several social and psychological problems for both the patient and carers. Feeding regimens may curtail social life, and sleep disruption may be a particular problem for patients on overnight feeding. Work or school may be disrupted by the feed regimen, but this should be avoided if possible. Patients may be unhappy at their inability to sit and enjoy meals with the rest of the family; they may also feel hungry if unable to eat anything by mouth. However, it should be emphasised that many patients on HEN can take small amounts of food by mouth and should be encouraged to do so.

The feeding regimen may be just one of a patient's needs: they may also require a number of medicines, oxygen, a urinary catheter, and have problems with faecal incontinence and mobility.

Drug administration

Many patients using enteral feeds also require medication, and complications can occur. In recent years the use of fine-bore tubes, different routes of feed administration, and the wide range of available feeds has made the use of drugs more complex. There are basically three main issues to consider in giving medicines to patients on enteral feeds: the route of administration, the formulation of the drug, and the possibility of interactions between the feed and the drug.

Route of administration

Some patients on enteral feeds can take medication by mouth, and this should be encouraged wherever possible. However, for those who cannot take medicines orally or cannot absorb them from the gastrointestinal tract, an alternative route will be required. Before considering an alternative route, however, the need for medication should be thoroughly reviewed. Not all of it may be indicated and the fewer drugs the patient is on, the less the chance of complications.

Various routes of administration may be considered in an enterally fed patient. Wherever possible, medication should not be given via the feeding tube. Intravenous administration may be used, but requires appropriately trained staff, is potentially prone to complications and tends to be expensive. It is not therefore generally suitable for patients being fed at home. Other routes include buccal and sublingual (e.g. buccal prochlorperazine, buccal or sublingual glyceryl trinitrate, or sublingual nifedipine), transdermal (e.g. glyceryl trinitrate patches), rectal (e.g. aspirin, bisacodyl, carbamazepine, and diclofenac suppositories) or nebulisation (e.g. salbutamol). Subcutaneous or intramuscular injections offer further options.

Sometimes it may be better to change the medicine to a similar one that can be given by a different route. For example, buccal prochlorperazine could be used instead of oral metoclopramide, rectal bisacodyl instead of oral laxatives, and piroxicam melt instead of oral non-steroidal anti-inflammatory drugs (NSAIDs).

When other routes of administration are unavailable, medication may be given via the feeding tube. The size and placement of the tube affect the administration of drugs via the tube: fine-bore tubes are unsuitable for the administration of thick liquids and dispersible tablets. Where medication and feeds are given via the same tube, an 8 gauge tube or larger is normally recommended, as this reduces the risk of blockage.

There are more likely to be problems with the absorption of medication when patients are fed postpylorically (i.e. into the duodenum or jejunum rather than the stomach), because the tube may extend into an area of the intestine beyond the absorption site of the drug. Alternative routes of administration should therefore be used when possible. Drugs whose absorption may be compromised by postpyloric feeding include cephalexin, digoxin, ketoconazole and phenytoin.

The practice of adding drugs directly to enteral feeds, rather than via the feeding tube but separate from the feed, should be avoided. This is because there is a risk of microbial contamination of the feed, difficulty in predicting the effect of the drug on the stability of the feed, difficulty in predicting potential drug interactions, and an increased risk of tube blockage.

Formulation

Liquids

The formulation of choice for a drug administered via a feeding tube is generally a liquid. Information on drugs available as liquids can be found in the *British National Formulary* and from 'specials' manufacturing units, both pharmaceutical companies and local NHS special units.

Although liquid preparations are preferred, difficulties can still occur. For example, many liquids are available only in paediatric strengths, necessitating the use of very large volumes to achieve adequate doses. In addition, not all liquids are suitable for administration via an enteral tube. Lansoprazole suspension, for example, is too viscous; diazepam may be adsorbed on to the plastic tubing; and Augmentin suspensions should be diluted to half strength to avoid 'caking'.

Sorbitol is frequently added to sugar-free preparations and its high osmolality can cause diarrhoea, bloating and stomach cramps. Liquids with a high osmolality or high sorbitol content should be avoided, particularly if the patient requires several medicines. Preparations of high osmolality can sometimes be diluted, although routine dilution is not recommended because of potential stability problems.

In general, suspensions or elixirs should be used in preference to syrups, but in some cases parenteral formulations may be the only suitable or available liquid preparation. However, they are expensive and are suitable for short-term use only.

Tablets and capsules

If a suitable liquid preparation is not available, an alternative is a soluble or dispersible tablet. However, if there is no other alternative, ordinary tablets may have to be crushed or the contents of capsules emptied and flushed down the tube (Table 10.3). Tablets should be crushed to a fine powder using a pestle and mortar or tablet crusher and then mixed with water. Tap water is usually suitable unless the drug is known to chelate with ions in tap water (e.g. ciprofloxacin), in which case sterile water should be used.

However, not all tablets are suitable for crushing (e.g. enteric-coated tablets). Crushing sustained- or modified-release preparations destroys their slow-release properties and may compromise therapeutic efficacy. Cytotoxic agents or other preparations with carcinogenic or teratogenic potential (e.g. hormones and prostaglandin analogues)

Table 10.3 Administration of medicines via enteral feeding tubes

- Crush tablets (with a pestle and mortar or tablet crusher) or open capsules and mix with 10–15 mL of tap water (5–10 mL for children). Dispersible tablets should also be mixed with 10–15 mL of tap water. A liquid preparation should be shaken before use
- Rinse the pestle and mortar or tablet crusher and flush all washings down the tube
- Draw up the prepared medication in a 50 mL needleless oral syringe (the use of smaller syringes causes the build-up of too much pressure in the tube)
- Flush the tube with 30 mL of tap water (sterile water for jejunal tubes) before administration of the medicine and before resuming the feed
- Give each drug separately. Do not mix any drugs prior to administration. Flush the tube with 5–10 mL of tap water in between each medicine. Flush the syringe with water in between drawing up each medicine

should not be crushed because of the risk to the person carrying out the crushing. Buccal or sublingual preparations should not be crushed and administered via feeding tubes because they are designed to bypass the gastrointestinal tract and avoid first-pass metabolism. Chewable tablets and pancreatic enzymes should also not be crushed.

Hard gelatin capsules can be emptied and the contents mixed with a suitable diluent. However, some capsules contain pellets or enteric-coated granules (e.g. omeprazole and lansoprazole) designed to be given intact, and these are not suitable for administration via fine-bore tubes. The contents of some soft gel capsules (e.g. chloral hydrate and nifedipine) may be withdrawn and flushed down the tube. If in any doubt, it is best to contact manufacturers for specialist advice.

Drug interactions with enteral feeds

When drugs and feeds are administered via the same tube, the potential for interactions and tube blockage increases. These difficulties can usually be prevented by careful timing of medication administration in relation to feeding. For patients on continuous feeding regimens this may require stopping the feed briefly, which can reduce the total amount of feed administered in a 24-hour period. The nutrient content of the feed and/or the rate of feed administration may therefore need to be increased. When breaks in feeding are required, the drug should be chosen so that it can be given as infrequently as possible (e.g. once or twice daily). If the patient is being fed overnight only, drugs can be given during the day.

Drugs can interfere with the absorption or metabolism of one or more nutrients in the feed. For example, tetracyclines taken at the same time as an enteral feed can chelate with calcium, magnesium, iron, and zinc and other di- and trivalent cations, so reducing the absorption of both the minerals and the antibiotic. Sucralfate binds with proteins in enteral feeds and can cause tube blockage, and it is recommended that the feed is stopped one hour before and resumed one hour after the drug is given. However, if sucralfate is being given for the prophylaxis of stress ulceration (i.e. 1 g six times daily), this could result in the loss of 12 hours' feeding time.

Pharmacists will be aware that the presence of food in the stomach can reduce the absorption of some drugs. This also applies to enteral feeds. For example, captopril, flucloxacillin, theophylline and verapamil are usually administered on an empty stomach as they are better tolerated or more bioavailable. For patients on continuous feeding regimens the feed should be stopped 15–30 minutes before administration of the drug to facilitate gastric emptying. The feed is resumed 30–60 minutes later to allow time for drug absorption.

Enteral feeds can interfere with drug metabolism. For example, warfarin metabolism is antagonised by vitamin K, a common component in enteral feeds. Phenytoin has reduced plasma levels if given with an enteral feed. The best way to minimise the risk of this interaction for patients on continuous feeding is to stop the feed two hours before giving the drug and resume it two hours later. Phenytoin levels should be monitored regularly, and it is important to ensure that the drug is given at exactly the same time and in the same way every day. This enables appropriate interpretation of serum drug levels. A photograph of a patient receiving home enteral nutrition is shown in Figure 10.4.

Monitoring and follow-up of HEN

As soon as enteral tube feeding is initiated, patients and carers need to understand its administration. More specifically, patients need to be instructed on the operation of the pump (if applicable), the use of giving sets, care of the equipment, including the importance of good hygiene, flushing the tube, and providing and collecting feeds and equipment. All patients and carers should have a list of contacts, both in the community (e.g. the GP, district nurse, community dietitian and pharmacist) and at the hospital. The availability of a troubleshooting service in case of problems is important.

Arrangements for monitoring should also be clarified. The patient will require routine monitoring at regular intervals, to assess the response to treatment and if necessary to re-evaluate treatment goals. It is important to check that the feeding regimen and feeding route remain appropriate and to ensure that complications are minimised. The ability of patients and carers to cope with the treatment should also be assessed.

Monitoring can be conducted at home or in the hospital. It involves checking the body weight and other anthropometric measurements (e.g. triceps skinfold thickness, mid-arm circumference and grip strength), biochemistry (e.g. urea and electrolytes) and state of hydration. The feeding regimen and the condition of the feeding tube should also be reviewed. For patients with a gastrostomy, the condition of the skin surrounding the stoma should also be assessed.

Frequency of monitoring will depend on the age and diagnosis of the patient, their stability and nutritional status, and the need of the carer for professional support. Depending on local arrangements, adults

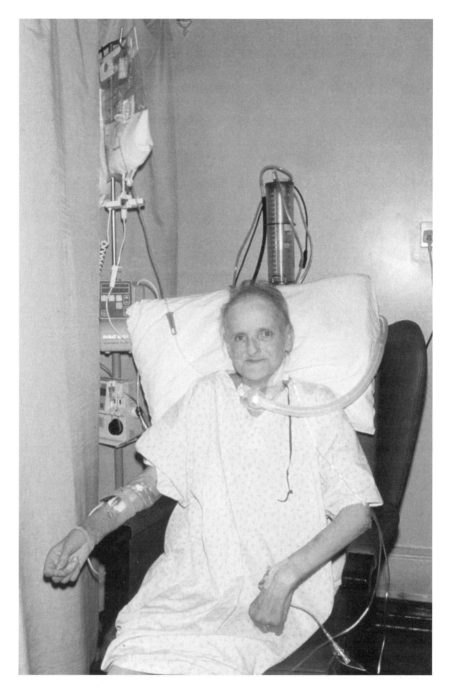

Figure 10.4 A patient receiving home enteral nutrition. (Courtesy of Centre for Pharmacy Postgraduate Education.)

recently discharged from hospital, those who are malnourished, or those with recent changes to the feeding regimen or abnormal biochemistry may be monitored once a month. However, a patient well-established on a stable feeding regimen may require monitoring once every three or four months. Infants and young children are generally monitored more frequently.

Role of the pharmacist

Pharmacists working in the community can have a significant role in helping to reduce the problems associated with undernutrition by keeping an eye on patients they know to be vulnerable. This includes older people, and particularly those on multiple-drug regimens or those who have recently been bereaved and live alone. Older people living in care homes and those who have recently had surgery or been in hospital for any reason may be at risk; these are all people with whom community pharmacists deal every day.

If a person is suspected of being at nutritional risk, pharmacists can ask questions about issues such as recent and past eating habits, changes in body weight, ability to shop, cook, swallow and chew, and whether the person has been subject to psychological stress (e.g. bereavement). If the pharmacy has a weighing machine it is also a good idea to weigh the person to get an indication of the body mass index (BMI) (weight (kg)/height $(m)^2$). If the BMI is less than 20, the person is underweight and could be at risk of malnutrition. Such people should be referred to a GP because they may need nutritional support.

Improving the intake of normal food is the first-choice intervention and can be achieved in a variety of ways, depending on the patient's problem. Offering small tasty snacks on a frequent basis can be helpful for patients who feel daunted by large meals; for those with sore mouths, bland puréed foods can be a useful option, together with the avoidance of foods that are too acidic or too dry. The addition of high-calorie ingredients (e.g. cream and butter) to normal foods can help to improve energy intake. Nutritional supplements containing fat, carbohydrate or both are available for addition to ordinary foods (see Chapter 8). A nutritional supplement in the form of a sip feed can be given (Table 10.4), or a combination of these approaches may be required to achieve adequate oral intake. However, in some situations the patient will benefit from being fed by tube directly into the gastrointestinal tract.

Table 10.4 Common examples of sip feeds, puddings and fortified soups approved by ACBS guidelines

Calshake	Fortijuice
Clinutren ISO	Fortimel
Clinutren 1.5	Fortisip
Clinutren Dessert	Fortisip Multifibre
Complan Ready to Drink	Fresubin
Enlive	Fresubin Energy Fibre
Enrich	Maxisorb
Enrich Plus	Provide Xtra
Ensure	QuickCal
Ensure Plus	Resource Dessert Energy, Protein Extra
Formance	and Shake
Forticreme	Scandishake
Fortifresh	Vitasavoury

Further reading

Elia M (ed.) (2000). *Guidelines for detection and management of malnutrition.* Malnutrition Advisory Group. (A standing committee of BAPEN).

Useful addresses

British Association of Parenteral and Enteral Nutrition (BAPEN)
PO Box 922
Maidenhead
Berkshire SL6 4SH
www.bapen.org.uk

British Pharmaceutical Nutrition Group
www.bpng.co.uk

Patients on Intravenous and Nasogastric Nutrition Therapy (PINNT)
PO Box 3126
Christchurch
Dorset BH23 2XS
Tel: 01202 481625
www.pinnt.com

11

Dialysis at home

Eileen J Laughton

Dialysis and transplantation are the specific forms of treatment for end-stage renal disease (ESRD; end-stage renal failure, ESRF; end-stage kidney failure). It has been estimated that 80–100 people per million of the population develop ESRD each year, and the numbers are increasing with the increasing age of the population. In terms of total numbers, there are almost 200 000 people in the UK receiving treatment for ESRD. For most the ideal solution is transplantation but, as demand for donor organs far outstrips the supply (see Organ donor cards, below), dialysis remains the only satisfactory alternative.

The options for a patient awaiting renal transplantation are peritoneal dialysis and haemodialysis. These techniques provide an alternative means of carrying out the healthy kidney's function of haemofiltration, which is vital to the removal of waste materials from the body. In the UK, approximately 50% of patients on dialysis are treated by continuous ambulatory peritoneal dialysis (CAPD); this figure is higher than in other countries, where patient choice is not so limited. When corrected for various parameters CAPD gives patient survival that is broadly comparable to that of haemodialysis, but this estimate is controversial.

It is unlikely that community pharmacists will have a significant input into the care and management of patients who are undergoing dialysis at home, as the majority of patients receive their dialysis equipment and fluids direct from a manufacturer or from the local hospital pharmacy. However, patients who have been selected for one of the forms of dialysis may have been and continue to be regular visitors to the community pharmacy with prescriptions necessary for the satisfactory management of their condition (e.g. for the treatment of hypertension beforehand and the supply of low-protein foods after starting dialysis). A pharmacy may be located close to a renal unit, and it is essential that pharmacists should be aware of the theoretical and practical aspects of the treatment the patient is receiving and the problems that may be encountered.

Classification and symptoms of ESRD

Chronic renal failure progresses over a period of many years and is defined as a steady, irreversible decline in the efficient working of the kidney owing to the slow destruction of renal tissue. It can be classified in terms of the creatinine clearance as follows:

- Mild: creatinine clearance   20–50 mL/min
- Moderate: creatinine clearance   10–20 mL/min
- Severe: creatinine clearance   <10 mL/min.

According to UK Renal Association guidelines, renal replacement therapy is indicated at the onset of ESRD. At this time, the creatinine clearance falls below 10 mL/min (i.e. less than 10% of normal, equivalent to a sustained serum creatinine concentration of >500 µmol/L); this value is not absolute, however, and symptoms should also be taken into account. Urea kinetic modelling may also be useful in determining whether treatment is necessary.

In the early stages there may be very few outward signs of the illness. Urine production does not decrease significantly, but in fact may paradoxically increase and be noticed by the patient when sleep is disturbed by the need for night-time micturition. This increase reflects the reduced ability of the kidneys to concentrate urine.

Other signs of chronic renal failure may develop insidiously, and patients may not recognise the deterioration in their health until the disease has advanced considerably. The commonest symptom is a general feeling of tiredness, which may be related to the presence of anaemia and the build-up of urea in the blood. Irritability may be a consequence of tiredness, as relatively simple tasks become major obstacles to be overcome. Dyspnoea on exertion may be noticeable and may be caused by anaemia, hypertension and, in later stages, emphysema.

In advanced stages of the disease, the skin may appear muddy and become dry and flaked. This is a result of reduced production of the keratin layer of the epidermis and decreased functioning of the sebaceous glands. The colour of the skin may darken owing to increased melanin production. Endocrine function is also disturbed. Libido may be reduced and impotence may develop in men. Dysmenorrhoea and menstrual irregularities may aggravate reduced sexual interest in women. The presence of urea in saliva and gastric secretions may affect the sense of taste and produce ammoniacal breath, reduced appetite and occasional vomiting. Cramps, particularly at night, may be associated with spasmodic tics which severely hamper manual dexterity. The development of oedema may be particularly noticeable in the ankles and face.

Bone disease may occur, especially in children and young adults. This is due to the reduced production of the active form of vitamin D (1,25-dihydroxycolecalciferol or calcitriol) and increased levels of parathyroid hormone. The effect of oversecretion of parathormone is to increase the transfer of calcium from bone into the blood. Levels of calcium in bone are further reduced by its exchange for the excess hydrogen ions (metabolic acidosis) that occur in the circulation as a result of reduced renal excretion. Hypercalcaemia has further consequences. Calcium phosphate deposition may occur in joints and in the periarticular tissues, producing gout-like symptoms.

In the final stages of the disease, severe intractable pruritus, tingling sensations in the feet, legs and hands, and hiccups may develop. Dermatological symptoms are caused by paraesthesia, thought to be due to the presence of urea in the nerve endings. Finally, the patient may slip into unconsciousness, have a seizure, or develop severe pain in the chest due to pericarditis.

Causes of ESRD

Glomerulonephritis

Glomerulonephritis accounts for over 10% of the patients with ESRD in Europe. It is an umbrella term serving to describe the end-result of a number of clinical syndromes (see below). Many cases of glomerulonephritis are due to the production of antigen–antibody complexes generated as a result of infection in other parts of the body (e.g. as the result of an autoimmune disease). In their passage through the kidneys, these complexes are filtered less efficiently than other materials and gradually accumulate in the glomerulus. Their presence can provoke an inflammatory response (nephritis), which leads to damage to the glomerular membranes and the subsequent loss of protein and blood in the urine. If inflammation is temporary, little scar tissue will be laid down. However, in the event of prolonged deposition of these complexes, inflammation is chronic and scar tissue gradually replaces the healthy tissue, not only of the glomerulus but also of the kidney tubule.

Acute nephritis produces haematuria and intense inflammation. The volume of urine passed is reduced and, on continued fluid intake, the face becomes swollen and hypertension develops. Pyrexia may occur, especially in the presence of infection. The most common causative organisms are streptococci, but with the introduction of the penicillins the incidence of acute nephritis has fallen dramatically. In most cases acute nephritis is a self-limiting condition, although it may take up to 12 months for proteinuria and microscopic haematuria to clear completely. Only in a minority of cases does the condition progress to nephrotic syndrome and renal failure.

Recurrent haematuria, which is more common in young males than in other groups, may also be a complication of acute sore throat or upper respiratory tract infection. The urine is coloured red or brown owing to the presence of blood, although its volume remains normal and hypertension is usually absent. Immunoglobulin A (IgA) antibodies may be found in the glomeruli on biopsy, and may occur in the secretions of the body (e.g. in saliva and gastric secretions). If proteinuria also develops there may be a gradual decline towards renal failure (over 20–30 years).

A decreased output of urine is characteristic of the nephrotic syndrome. The urine is frothy, owing to the presence of large quantities of protein (mainly albumin) whose loss from the blood leads to the accumulation of fluid in the tissues. Gross swelling may be apparent around the face, ankles, feet, abdomen and genitals, and may be severe enough to immobilise the patient. Renal biopsy invariably shows significant structural damage to the glomeruli whereby the permeability of the glomerular basement membrane is increased. Diuretics may reduce the degree of oedema, and long-term management may require the introduction of foods low in sodium but high in protein.

Glomerulonephritis may also be a consequence of systemic disease, such as systemic lupus erythematosus (SLE), a connective tissue autoimmune disorder which mainly affects adolescent and young adult women. Antibodies present in the circulation but normally quiescent react against tissue components (e.g. DNA) and form complexes which are deposited in the kidneys, brain, eyes and joints. The outward manifestations of the disease are skin rash, commonly occurring as a butterfly rash over the bridge of the nose and cheeks, and arthralgia. Rarely, glomerulonephritis may be the initial symptom, and may cause rapid deterioration to uraemia and renal failure.

Other less common systemic precursors of glomerulonephritis include Henoch–Schönlein purpura, Goodpasture's syndrome, polyarteritis, Wegener's granulomatosis and scleroderma.

Pyelonephritis

Pyelonephritis is a term that describes involvement of the kidney in a urinary tract infection. Reflux of urine from the bladder to the kidneys (vesicoureteric reflux) in association with infection is a potent source of pyelonephritis and may result in scarring of the tissue and subsequent deterioration to chronic renal failure.

The presence of calculi in the renal tract may lead to infection. Most calculi are formed of calcium salts (commonly phosphate and oxalate), and the presence of small sharp-edged stones may give rise to considerably more intense symptoms than larger smoother stones. Characteristic symptoms include renal colic (which may be so severe as to cause vomiting) and haematuria caused by the stone being lodged within the ureter.

Cystic diseases of the kidney may produce pyelonephritis. Polycystic renal disease is the commonest inherited kidney disease and produces an enlarged kidney, with much of the normal tissue replaced by fibrous tissue and cysts. Recurrent or persistent pyelonephritis may be one of the signs whose investigation leads to the identification of ESRD. Polycystic renal disease tends to develop at 30–40 years of age and progresses to ESRD over a period of 10–15 years; secondary hypertension is common.

Pyelonephritis may also accompany prostatitis and gynaecological disorders.

Vascular disease and hypertension

The link between hypertension and renal function is well documented. Kidney disease can lead to high blood pressure, which in turn can further damage the kidneys, setting up a vicious circle of events which, if untreated, will invariably result in renal failure. The kidney diseases that commonly cause hypertension are glomerulonephritis, vesicoureteric reflux and polycystic renal disease. On the other hand, renovascular hypertension may be caused by renal artery stenosis due to fibrosis or the laying down of atheroma. This develops in the absence of significant renal impairment through activation of the renin–angiotensin–aldosterone axis.

Diabetes mellitus

Diabetes mellitus is the commonest cause of ESRD in Europe and the USA. Mild forms of renal disease may manifest as proteinuria, but in severe cases the nephrotic syndrome may develop. In both, a mean time of 12 years has been shown to elapse between the onset of proteinuria and the development of uraemia and renal failure. The presence of high concentrations of glucose in the urine provides an ideal medium for the growth of microorganisms, and pyelonephritis may be a further complication in the onset of renal failure.

Analgesic abuse

Ingestion of large quantities of analgesics (especially those containing aspirin or other non-steroidal anti-inflammatory agents) has been linked with the development of chronic renal failure through renal papillary necrosis or chronic interstitial nephritis. The drugs may be taken as self-medication or be prescribed to treat another condition (e.g. arthritis).

Non-specific measures in the management of ESRD

Treatment of hypertension

Many patients have been on long-term antihypertensive therapy before ESRD develops. Patients may also have been advised of dietary and life-style adjustments necessary to supplement the drug regimen. Blood pressure may be reduced by the restriction of salt intake to the equivalent of about 80–100 mmol of sodium per day. Eliminating foods that contain large quantities of salt and eating foods without further salt additions may be beneficial. Patients may also benefit from relaxation techniques (e.g. meditation) that reduce the effects of stress on their lifestyle.

Protein restriction has been advocated, but its benefits are not universally accepted. Historically, the restriction of protein to about 20 g/day in conjunction with a high-carbohydrate diet was shown to reduce the levels of urea and creatinine and relieve symptoms of renal failure. However, the low palatability and poor energy content of commercially available protein-restricted diets often led to patients becoming severely malnourished. Less strict reductions are now recommended for patients in the early stages of renal failure: the daily protein intake is kept to 0.8–1.0 g per kg body weight (based on the ideal) daily, and is supplied from animal sources (e.g. meat, fish, eggs and milk).

Other measures

One benefit of a low protein intake is the concurrent reduction in phosphate levels. This helps to keep the patient free from bone and joint complications. If levels of phosphate are considered too high, intestinal phosphate-binding agents (e.g. calcium salts or sevelamer) can be administered.

Potassium levels may also require restriction. If the patient is producing adequate quantities of urine, potassium levels may remain within normal limits. Even when urinary output is reduced, compensatory mechanisms operate to increase the urinary concentration of potassium. Despite this mechanism, however, build-up of potassium may still occur, particularly in the later stages of kidney failure, necessitating dietary restriction. Foods which are high in potassium and should be restricted include the following:

Dates, figs, prunes	Toffee, chocolate, fudge
Other dried fruit	Crisps, chips, and other forms of potato
Avocados	Fruit juices
Oranges	Coffee, cocoa, Horlicks
Bananas	Evaporated and condensed milk
Mushrooms	Strong ale
Beetroot	Tomato ketchup
Rhubarb	Meat and yeast extracts
Liquorice	Salt substitutes

High-fibre cereals are also high in potassium, but their benefits (avoidance of constipation) are considered to outweigh any effect on potassium balance. There is some evidence that lowering plasma cholesterol and the use of low-fat diets is beneficial; a daily dietary fat intake of 30–35% of the total energy intake is recommended (this may be increased in a protein-restricted diet and should be mainly in the form of polyunsaturated fats). Because a protein- and phosphate-restricted diet may lead to the development of hypocalcaemia, calcium supplements may be useful.

Books and leaflets suggesting recipes and foods suitable for ESRD patients are available from kidney patient support organisations (see below).

Drug restrictions

The kidney is the major route of excretion of many drugs, and the ESRD patient is particularly susceptible to the build-up of drugs in the body that results from reduced renal function. A comprehensive list of these drugs and a discussion of the problems of drug administration in renal failure are included in the BNF, which should be consulted for current information. Table 11.1 summarises some of the commoner drugs whose use may be associated with problems in varying stages of kidney failure (the requirement for modification of maintenance dose is achieved by increasing the interval between each dose of the drug, or by reducing the size of each individual dose).

The principles of dialysis

In very simple terms, the kidney acts as a filter to remove waste materials and excess water from the body and conserves essential components necessary for the homoeostatic maintenance of health. The initial process of ultrafiltration of blood components occurs in the glomerulus. Water and simple solutes are removed from the plasma and enter the glomerulus, with the result that the concentrations of solutes in the

Table 11.1 Drug modifications required in varying degrees of ESRD

Drug	Stage of failure	Action
ACE inhibitors	Mild/moderate	Adjust initial dose and monitor response
Aciclovir	Mild	Reduce i.v. dose
	Moderate/severe	Reduce dose
Ampicillin	Moderate/severe	Reduce dose
Atenolol	Moderate	Reduce dose
Azathioprine	Severe	Reduce dose
Bumetanide	Moderate	May need high doses
Cephalosporins	Moderate/severe	Reduce dose
Chlorpropamide	Mild/moderate/severe	Avoid
Co-trimoxazole	Moderate	Reduce dose
Diazepam	Severe	Reduce initial dose
Digoxin	Mild	Reduce dose
Furosemide	Moderate	May need high doses
Gentamicin	Mild	Reduce dose
Heparin	Severe	Reduce dose or avoid
Hydralazine	Mild	Reduce dose
Losartan	Moderate/severe	Halve initial dose
Metoclopramide	Moderate/severe	Reduce dose
Morphine		see Opioids
Nitrofurantoin	Mild	Avoid
Opioids	Moderate/severe	Reduce dose or avoid
Pentazocine	Severe	Reduce dose or avoid
Phenobarbitone	Severe	Avoid large doses
Prochlorperazine	Severe	Start with small dose
Simvastatin	Moderate/severe	Caution with doses >10 mg daily
Tetracyclines	Mild	Avoid (except doxycycline and minocycline)
Valsartan	Moderate/severe	Halve initial dose

filtrate are essentially the same as in the blood plasma. Under normal circumstances, protein does not pass through the glomerular membrane in any significant quantities. As the filtrate passes along the tubule of the nephron, solutes are selectively reabsorbed. In the proximal convoluted tubule, about two-thirds of the sodium ions, potassium ions and water, about half the urea, all of the amino acids and glucose, and the tiny quantities of protein that have leaked through the glomerular membrane are reabsorbed. Sodium, bicarbonate, calcium and chloride are reabsorbed in the proximal and distal convoluted tubules; potassium and uric acid are reabsorbed in the proximal tubule and resecreted in the distal tubule. A further 20% of the water content of the filtrate is reabsorbed in the distal tubule. Creatinine is predominantly filtered from the blood at the glomerulus and is not reabsorbed in the tubules. The measure of creatinine clearance is therefore taken as an indication of the functioning capacity of the kidney. Urea, one of the end-products of the metabolism of protein, is usually completely filtered and eliminated from the kidney, but is a less useful measure of renal function as the rate of production varies and about 40–50% is reabsorbed.

In renal failure, artificial means must be created to carry out the process of ultrafiltration. The basis for all forms of dialysis is the passage of small solute molecules in the blood down a concentration gradient and across a semipermeable membrane into a dialysing fluid. The technique was originally tried in the early part of the 1900s, but only became used on a large scale in the 1960s (haemodialysis) and 1970s (continuous ambulatory peritoneal dialysis). The introduction of heparin in 1926 and the development of polymer science in the 1960s, permitting the manufacture of long-lasting inert cannulas made of polytetrafluoroethylene (PTFE), are responsible for this wider use of dialysis.

New technology has also made possible internal junctions (fistulas) for joining arteries and veins directly, or internal woven plastics such as Dacron can be used to connect arteries and veins under the skin. New membranes have also been developed, but the basic principles remain unchanged.

Peritoneal dialysis

Patients undergoing peritoneal dialysis constitute the largest group undergoing positive treatment for ESRD at home. The principle of peritoneal dialysis is based on contact between a dialysing fluid and the peritoneum. Briefly, fluid is pumped into the peritoneal cavity (which normally contains about 100 mL of fluid but can expand to hold up to

5 L) and is left *in situ* to dialyse and extract water and small molecules across the peritoneum into the bloodstream. The fluid is then drained from the cavity and the cycle repeated.

The technique can be classified as continuous ambulatory peritoneal dialysis (CAPD) or automated peritoneal dialysis (APD). In CAPD the dialysis fluid is in continuous contact with the peritoneal membrane and the patient is able to walk around; in APD, the contact of the dialysis fluid with the peritoneal membrane is intermittent and the patient remains connected to a machine during dialysis.

The peritoneum is the membrane that lines the inner surface of the abdominal cavity. It is composed of mesothelial cells from which tiny projections, the microvilli, arise, unevenly distributed over the surface of the membrane. The surface area of the peritoneum is between 1.7 and 2 m², approximately equivalent to that of the skin. The peritoneum has a profuse capillary network, and it is through these capillaries that the process of ultrafiltration occurs.

Ultrafiltration is facilitated by the presence in the dialysis fluid of high concentrations of an osmotic agent, usually glucose. The osmotic gradient between the peritoneal and intravascular fluid compartments acts as the driving force for the passage of water across the peritoneal membrane into the peritoneal cavity. The concentration of glucose in the dialysis solution is selected according to the amount of fluid the patient needs to remove.

Fluid is introduced into the peritoneal cavity through a permanent indwelling sterile silastic rubber catheter (most commonly a straight Tenckhoff type), which is distinguished from other catheters by the presence of many fine holes in one side of the indwelling portion. The catheter is kept in position by the ingrowth of fibrous tissue from the abdominal wall into two Dacron cuffs situated along the catheter.

An external connector is used to connect the dialysis container and its tubing. The exit site of the catheter from the abdominal wall can be cleaned and covered with a dressing, or left open to the atmosphere to allow showering and drying, which may reduce the risk of bacterial infection.

CAPD

There has been an upsurge in the number of patients treated with CAPD since the early 1980s, with approximately 50% of all dialysis patients using this method by the mid-1990s. It is the most popular method of treatment for new patients, possibly because choice is limited by the shortage of donors for kidney transplantation and by the lack of development of hospital and home facilities for the treatment of patients with haemodialysis. A patient selected for CAPD treatment is mobile (hence the term ambulatory) and can be treated at home, and no large capital outlay is required to establish the treatment. It has also been established as the treatment of choice for children and for patients with diabetes, and it may be preferred when there is cardiovascular instability or if there are problems with venous access.

In CAPD, typically, 2–3 L of dialysis fluid are infused under gravity into the peritoneal cavity via a permanent peritoneal catheter (Figure 11.1). The solution is warmed to body temperature before administration,

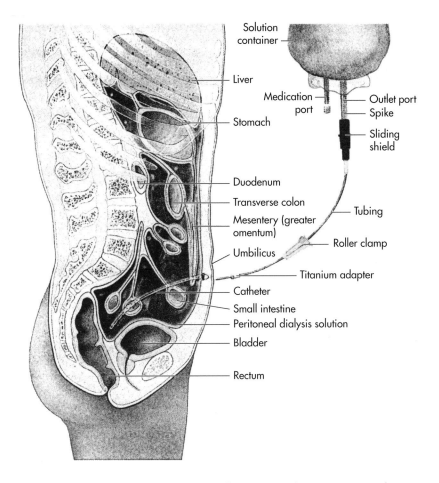

Figure 11.1 CAPD solution exchange: infusion procedure. (Courtesy of Baxter Healthcare Ltd.)

but it is imperative that a microwave oven is NOT used for this purpose as it may cause rupture of the bag, caramelisation of the glucose or deterioration of the structure of the bag. Three to five exchanges are made per day, in which the fluid in the peritoneal cavity is drained into an empty bag (Figure 11.2) and then replaced by fresh fluid. A Y- (disconnect; flush-before-fill) system is now used to join the catheter to the tubing leading from the bag containing the dialysis fluid and to the drainage bag, rather than the older type of system shown in Figures 11.1 and 11.2. This has removed the need for the patient to have the plastic bag attached all day.

The concentration of glucose in the peritoneal dialysis solution determines the solution's osmolality (and so determines the transfer of fluid across the membrane), and is selected according to how much fluid the patient is required to lose. Most commonly, a solution containing

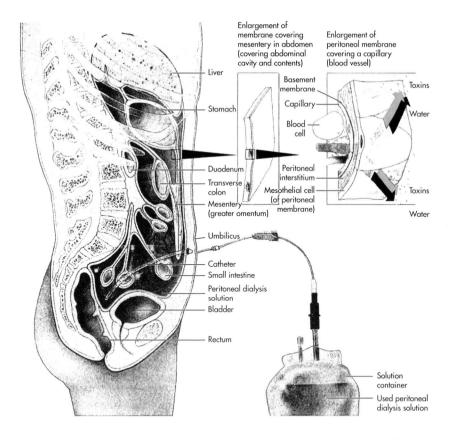

Figure 11.2 CAPD solution exchange: draining procedure. (Courtesy of Baxter Healthcare Ltd.)

1.36% anhydrous glucose (equivalent to 1.5% glucose monohydrate) is used; solutions containing 2.27% and 3.86% anhydrous glucose are also available. Improvements in peritoneal dialysis fluids have reduced the calcium content, with the aim of avoiding problems associated with raised serum calcium levels. An example of a peritoneal dialysis solution is given below. Each litre contains:

- Anhydrous glucose   13.6 g
- Sodium chloride   5.4 g
- Sodium lactate   4.5 g
- Calcium chloride   184 mg
- Magnesium chloride   51 mg.

This is expressed in millimoles per litre (mmol/L) as:

- Sodium   132
- Calcium   1.25
- Magnesium   0.25
- Chloride   95
- Lactate   40.

Other recent developments have included the formulation of a bicarbonate/lactate peritoneal dialysis solution, which is a more physiologically compatible solution that can correct acidosis and reduce the incidence of pain on infusion. The solution has a formula similar to that given above, but has a pH of 7.4 and contains 25 mmol/L of bicarbonate and 15 mmol/L of lactate. Peritoneal dialysis solutions containing amino acids have also been introduced to cater for malnourished ESRD patients, and the use of a solution containing icodextrin (a glucose polymer) instead of glucose in one exchange per day has allowed ultrafiltration to occur over an extended period, thereby avoiding the build-up of glucose degradation products. This is particularly useful for the long daytime dwell in some automated peritoneal dialysis regimens (see below).

An initial training programme for patients is given in the hospital renal unit, in which staff and other dialysis patients demonstrate the technique of exchange and the importance of sterile manipulations. The aseptic addition of drugs to the dialysis fluids may also be taught. Patients may be visited at home by a CAPD nursing sister until they are fully confident of carrying out their own CAPD.

Solutions can be supplied from the hospital pharmacy or direct from a distributor. Large storage areas are required in the home, as a patient's weekly requirement is normally 56 L. Other disposables (e.g.

sterile masks and surgical gloves), antiseptic solutions (for use around connecting systems) and dressings are required. These can be supplied at the same time as the fluids, or the patient can obtain supplies from the community pharmacy through the GP.

Advantages of CAPD

Patients can adapt CAPD exchanges to suit their lifestyle (e.g. one in the morning after rising, one at lunchtime, one in the early evening, and one before going to bed). In between exchanges, the patient is free to lead a virtually normal existence. Other advantages reflect the minimal disruption caused to the patient compared with haemodialysis. There is no need for the provision of special equipment or facilities, apart from storage, in the home (Figure 11.3). There may be less strain on the family because assistance from the partner, although advantageous, is not essential.

CAPD is less homoeostatically disruptive than other forms of dialysis. The dialysis solution is kept in contact with the blood for longer than in haemodialysis, and this results in less disturbance of the blood chemistry. The peritoneal membrane is more permeable to larger molecules than the haemodialysis membrane, and this may result in more effective removal of toxins whose presence can cause uraemia.

Hypertension and anaemia, particularly when associated with diabetes and polycystic renal disease, may be corrected by CAPD. This may be due to a reduction in the blood volume, which in some cases is severe enough to cause hypotension, and increased concentrations of haemoglobin. Reduction in the blood concentration of urea and the removal of erythropoietin inhibitors from the plasma have also been proposed as mechanisms responsible for these improvements. Intraperitoneal infusion of insulin can also be used to achieve good control of blood sugar in diabetic patients.

Dietary management can be less strict during peritoneal dialysis than in haemodialysis. Restrictions in sodium, refined carbohydrate and fluid intake may be necessary, as in all forms of renal failure (see above), to limit the development of obesity and hyperlipidaemia. Protein supplements may be required to replace the losses that occur, especially during peritonitis. Phosphate levels are controlled more effectively in patients undergoing CAPD than in those on intermittent peritoneal dialysis or haemodialysis. This in turn reduces the requirement for the use of phosphate-binding agents and may result in better control of renal osteodystrophy.

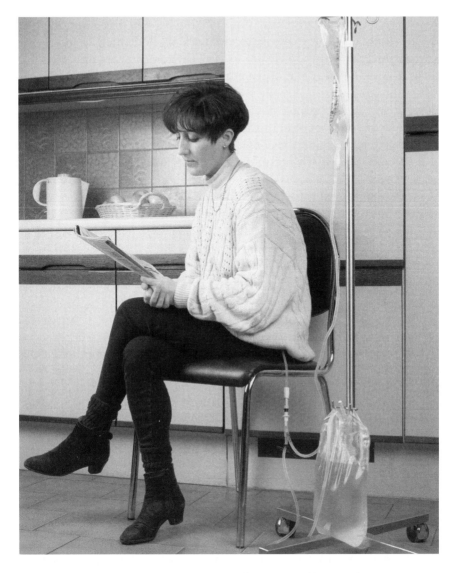

Figure 11.3 CAPD in progress. (Courtesy of Baxter Healthcare Ltd.)

Complications of CAPD

Peritonitis is the major complication of CAPD and is severe enough to warrant stopping the treatment and transferring the patient (when possible) to a haemodialysis programme. Peritonitis may be apparent from the discharge of cloudy fluid into the dialysis fluid collection bag. Symptoms of infection include abdominal pain, pyrexia, nausea and diarrhoea. Infection is commonly due to a breakdown of sterile technique in catheter manipulations, leakage of fluid from the catheter and the exit site, or infections at the exit site itself. The incidence of peritonitis has been reduced by the use of disconnect systems which incorporate a flush-before-fill procedure to remove microorganisms introduced by handling connectors. Further protection is gained by strict adherence to aseptic technique in catheter manipulations. Infection may also occur with intestinal flora introduced through the gut wall into the peritoneal cavity, usually in patients with bowel disease or perforation. Avoiding constipation is therefore important.

The method of treatment for peritoneal infection varies according to the causative organism. The initial step is usually the 'blind' administration of broad-spectrum antibiotic therapy (e.g. cefazolin and gentamicin) into the peritoneum to achieve a high local concentration, preferably without hospitalisation of the patient. Treatment is then tailored according to culture results: Gram-positive bacterial infections may require additional specific treatment for 14 or 21 days, but longer treatment may be necessary for Gram-negative organisms. If peritonitis persists, catheter removal and later replacement is considered.

Other complications may also arise. Obesity and hyperlipidaemia may occur because of the large quantities of glucose absorbed from the fluids infused into the peritoneum. This may increase the risk of cerebrovascular and cardiovascular problems, especially in the elderly.

Conversely, malnutrition may arise because of the loss of 6–12 g protein each day in the dialysate. In the presence of peritonitis, protein loss may be as high as 20 g/day. A positive nitrogen balance can be maintained by increasing protein intake in the diet (an intake of >1.2 g/kg ideal body weight daily is recommended by the UK Renal Association), or by supplementing nitrogen intake by adding amino acids to the peritoneal dialysis fluid.

Existing hernias may be aggravated in CAPD patients, often necessitating surgical correction. New hernias may also develop at the entry site of the intraperitoneal catheter, owing to disruption of the abdominal muscle wall. Back pain is a common problem and may be severe enough to warrant suspension of treatment.

Drug administration during CAPD

The kidney is the major route of excretion for drugs. In CAPD, significant elimination of drugs may occur into the dialysis fluid and the extent of elimination is increased in the presence of high-concentration glucose solutions. Pharmacists should therefore be aware of the drugs whose bioavailability profile may be altered in CAPD. Drugs of low protein-binding capacity, or with a low volume of distribution, whose major route of excretion is normally the kidneys, may be cleared across the peritoneal membrane in significant amounts. Examples of drugs in this category are vancomycin, the aminoglycosides and ceftazidime.

Drugs can also be added to the dialysis fluid as a means of systemic administration. The characteristics required for the attainment of adequate blood levels are high plasma protein binding and a large volume of distribution. Drugs that can be added to peritoneal dialysis fluids include antibiotics, mineral supplements and insulin. Cytotoxic drugs have also been administered by this route to treat ovarian cancer.

APD

In automated peritoneal dialysis (APD) a machine automatically controls the fill volume, dwell time and length of treatment. This technique encompasses a number of regimens, including intermittent peritoneal dialysis (IPD), and is most often carried out at home while the patient sleeps. A series of rapid exchanges are performed (an average of six exchanges of 1.5–6 L of dialysis fluid each night, dwelling in the peritoneal cavity for 30 minutes to 1 hour). In night-time intermittent peritoneal dialysis (NIPD) the peritoneum can remain dry through the day. However, more commonly, fluid from the final night-time exchange is left to dwell in the peritoneal cavity during the day.

The rapid overnight exchanges can be accompanied by one manual fluid exchange during the day, and the regimen may be optimised, if declining renal function dictates, by increasing the number of daytime exchanges. Another variation of APD, tidal peritoneal dialysis, is where only about 50–75% of the total volume of dialysate run into the peritoneal cavity is exchanged at each cycle (cycles are more frequent than in NIPD). This technique is suitable for those complaining of pain during each inflow or outflow.

At present, about 10% of peritoneal dialysis patients perform APD, but the proportion is steadily growing.

Advantages and disadvantages of APD

Modern APD machines are small, about the size of a video recorder (Figure 11.4). They are easily placed at a patient's bedside and can be transported if dialysis is to be carried out in a different place. Because of its flexibility, APD is generally suited to patients who work or study during the day and need to be free from the need for CAPD exchanges. It is also useful in those who need a carer to help perform their dialysis. The frequent exchanges of dialysis fluid makes APD particularly suitable for patients who are 'high transporters' (i.e. whose peritoneums transport solutes quickly).

APD is not suitable for patients with low-permeability peritoneal membranes (low transporters), as insufficient diffusion occurs during the short exchange cycle. Indeed, most patients tend to need an extra daytime exchange. The cost and space requirements of the large quantities of dialysis fluid needed for APD may also be a limiting factor when considering which dialysis technique to initiate.

Intermittent peritoneal dialysis (IPD) is now mostly restricted to a temporary form of dialysis (e.g. for those awaiting training for CAPD, for the management of fluid leaks, and in patients who have had abdominal surgery). It is also useful in debilitated or elderly patients with no vascular access, and in those who are otherwise unsuitable for haemodialysis or CAPD.

Home haemodialysis

Home haemodialysis is carried out by patients with ESRD, with minimal intervention from the hospital renal unit following an initial 6–12-week

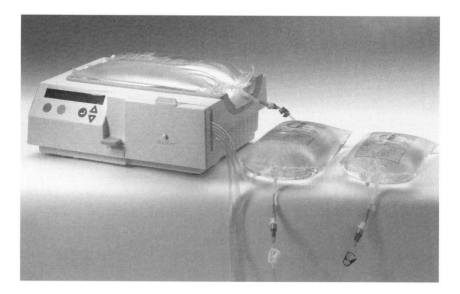

Figure 11.4 APD machine. (Courtesy of Baxter Healthcare Ltd.)

training programme. The principle of haemodialysis is described above. In brief, blood is removed from the body, combined with an anticoagulant, and passed over a semipermeable membrane across which solutes are transferred to and from a dialysis fluid. There is no requirement for the haemodialysis fluids to be sterile as the membrane does not permit the passage of bacteria.

Long-term vascular access for connecting the patient to the haemodialysis machine is usually achieved with an arteriovenous fistula, which ideally should be created well ahead of the anticipated start of dialysis. The fistula is created by the anastomosis of an artery and a vein, usually at the wrist or elbow. The vein becomes 'arterialised' over a period of time, permitting access by a wide-bore needle. At home, the needle is inserted into the vein by the patient, usually at the same point on each occasion and with the tip of the needle pointing into the flow of blood. Two needles may be inserted, with the blood-removing needle positioned distal to the blood-returning needle. Single-needle access, in which output and input is alternated every few seconds, is gaining in popularity; double-lumen needles are also available which allow a continuous flow of blood. Artificial fistulas may also be created using synthetic polymer materials (e.g. PTFE) to join an artery and a vein; this technique is more common in the USA than in the UK.

Emergency vascular access (e.g. if haemodialysis is suddenly needed while awaiting the maturation of a fistula) may be obtained with a temporary subclavian catheter inserted under local anaesthetic. Percutaneous catheters may also be inserted to provide permanent access for patients whose fistulae have failed or whose blood vessels are inadequate for fistula creation.

The exchange process uses a dialyser, which consists of a blood compartment and a dialysate compartment separated by a semipermeable membrane. Two designs are commonly used in the UK. The hollow-fibre type consists of thousands of tubular membranes inside which the blood flows in one direction with the dialysate flowing outside in the opposite direction. The parallel-plate type consists of a stack of membranes between which the dialysate flows (as in a sandwich). High performance is achieved by the contraflow of blood and dialysate. An increasing variety of semipermeable membranes has enabled clearance, fluid removal and biocompatibility to be tailored to an individual patient's needs. Membranes can be made from cellulose, modified cellulose or synthetic materials, and may be high flux (allowing clearance of solutes up to molecular weight (MW) 30 kDa) or low flux (less permeable to water and solutes, allowing passage of solutes up to MW 10 kDa).

The dialysis fluid is similar in composition to that used in CAPD, although acetate has traditionally been used in place of lactate to correct acidosis. This has largely been superseded by bicarbonate to give a more physiological solution, producing fewer metabolic disturbances. Large volumes of dialysis fluid are required (approximately 400 L/week) and fluid is passed through the dialyser at a high rate of 500 mL/min. The dialysis fluid is formed *in situ* by diluting a concentrate with purified water, warming this to body temperature and channelling it to the dialyser; bicarbonate, if used, is added as a separate concentrate or as a solid. Water must be pretreated with water softeners to remove calcium and magnesium; reverse osmosis, carbon filters and sediment filters may be necessary to remove microorganisms and ionic and particulate contaminants.

Ultrafiltration can be promoted by altering the pressure gradient across the semipermeable membrane in the dialysis machine. This leads to increased removal of urea and water from the blood and may be especially useful in patients with a large fluid overload. Most modern machines, however, use volumetric control to promote ultrafiltration, in which the inflow and outflow volumes are adjusted continuously.

Twenty-four-hour technical support is essential for home dialysis, and a large array of accessories is needed. Sterile solutions of heparin and normal saline and local anaesthetic injections are required to prepare for dialysis. Gauze swabs, antiseptic solutions and a variety of dressings and dressing packs are necessary for pre- and postdialysis care. Many of the items can be supplied for the home haemodialysis patient as part of the delivery of fluids. Some items can be obtained from the patient's GP and local community pharmacy.

Advantages of haemodialysis

The time required for dialysis each week has been steadily reduced over recent years by the use of more efficient dialysers. Patients can now be successfully managed by an average of four hours of haemodialysis three times a week (e.g. two evening sessions and one weekend session). Although many patients may prefer to shorten the time they are attached to the dialyser as much as possible (e.g. by using high-flux dialysers), overintensive haemodialysis can significantly reduce their wellbeing, particularly on the day after dialysis. This may be due to the rapid depletion of body fluids and solutes. Despite this effect, patients may feel less tied to their therapy than those using CAPD, although long-distance travel from the home may not be possible.

Disadvantages of haemodialysis

The physical requirements for haemodialysis in the home are considerable and the costs of initiating treatment may be prohibitive. Ideally, a spare room must be dedicated to the equipment, with appropriate plumbing and electricity installed. The support of the family is vital, although this may be restrictive for young patients who are preparing to set up home on their own. Large areas are required for the storage of accessories (e.g. disposable lines, fluids and drugs).

Hypotension may be a complication of haemodialysis, particularly if short, intensive periods of dialysis are used. The patient may complain of faintness, nausea and vomiting, and regular blood pressure measurements are recommended before, during and after the dialysis period (some machines perform this task automatically via a haematocrit and blood-volume measurement device, and alert the patient by an alarm). Back-flux may be permitted with high-performance membranes, increasing the likelihood of a pyrogenic reaction; higher-purity water is therefore required.

Dietary restrictions tend to fall between the often severe restrictions necessary for conservative management of ESRD and the milder restrictions considered appropriate for CAPD. Protein may be lost during dialysis, and the intake allowed may be greater than in conservative management (at least 1 g/kg ideal body weight daily is recommended), but still less than the normal dietary intake. Restriction of potassium, phosphate and sodium is also required, with sodium restriction being necessary to control blood pressure and thirst. Fluid restriction must be observed, as the production of urine between periods of connection to the haemodialysis unit is minimal. The kidneys cannot increase urine production if fluid intake increases, with the result that tissues may become oedematous (e.g. the lungs). Compliance with a fluid-restricted diet tends to be low; a daily intake of 500 mL of fluid plus the volume of the previous day's urine output is ideal.

Organ donor cards

All patients with ESRD should be considered for transplantation. Short-term survival of a cadaveric graft is 75–85% at one year and 70% at five years; the five-year survival increases to 90% with a living-related graft. The average wait for a graft, once the patient is accepted into the transplant programme in the UK, is four years.

For most people with ESRD the only chance of returning to a reasonably normal life is through kidney transplantation. Pharmacies often play a prominent role in displaying organ donor cards (Figure 11.5) and the use of these cards is considered briefly in this section. The removal of kidneys from deceased people in the UK is regulated by the Human Tissues Act 1961.

The organ donor card scheme allows a person's positive wish for donation to be known in the event of sudden death. Organs can then be removed without seeking permission from the nearest relatives, although in practice, if they are nearby they will still be approached.

The majority of organs come from cadaveric donation from patients who have suffered brainstem death and who are being maintained on a ventilator in an intensive care unit. The most appropriate organs for

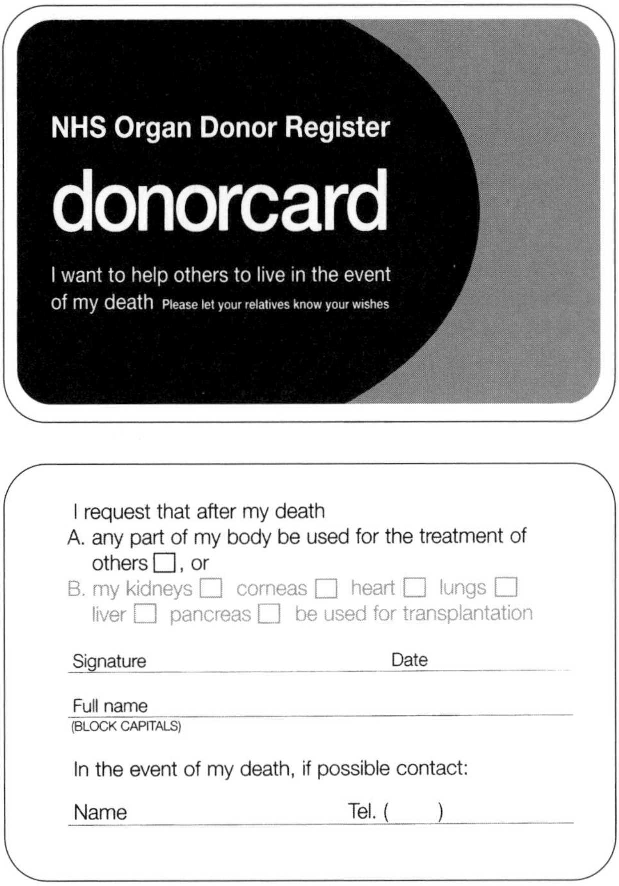

NHS Organ Donor Register

donorcard

I want to help others to live in the event of my death Please let your relatives know your wishes

I request that after my death
A. any part of my body be used for the treatment of others ☐, or
B. my kidneys ☐ corneas ☐ heart ☐ lungs ☐ liver ☐ pancreas ☐ be used for transplantation

Signature   Date

Full name
(BLOCK CAPITALS)

In the event of my death, if possible contact:

Name   Tel. (   )

Figure 11.5 Organ donor card. (Crown Copyright reproduced with permission from The Stationery Office Controller.)

transplantation come from young people fatally injured in road traffic accidents, or who have had a cerebral haemorrhage. Unsuitable donors include patients who have died with cancer (particularly in the presence of metastases), widespread infectious disease, heart failure and low blood pressure. Kidneys are rarely used from patients over 75 years of age. Transplantation is still not available for all who require it, and changes in the law, together with an increase in the number of intensive care beds in hospitals, may help increase the availability of donor organs from cadavers. It has been estimated that increasing the number of kidneys donated annually in the UK by approximately 20% would redress the shortfall. Ideally, patients should be made aware of the potential for transplants from living related (or non-related) donors. Recently, kidneys from asystolic (non-heart-beating) cadaveric patients have been used, in which ice-cold perfusion of the kidneys via an intra-aortic catheter is used to maintain the organs' viability. These developments, together with the concept of xenotransplantation (of kidneys from animals), however, remain controversial.

Further reading

Levy J, Morgan J, Brown E (eds) (2001). *Oxford Handbook of Dialysis*. Oxford: Oxford University Press.

Smith T (ed.) (1997). *Renal Nursing*. London: Baillière Tindall.

Stein A, Wild J (eds) (1999). *Kidney Failure Explained: Everything You Always Wanted to Know About Dialysis but Were Afraid to Ask*. London: Class Publishing.

The Renal Association (1997). *Treatment of Adult Patients with Renal Failure: Recommended Standards and Audit Measures*, 2nd edn. London: Royal College of Physicians.

Useful addresses

British Kidney Patient Association
Oakhanger Place
Bordon
Hants GU35 9JP
Tel: 01420 472021

National Kidney Federation
6 Stanley Street
Worksop
Notts S81 7HX
Tel: 01909 487795

National Kidney Research Fund
Kings Chambers
Priestgate
Peterborough PE1 1FG
Tel: 01733 704678
www.nkrf.org.uk

Renal Association
Royal College of Physicians
11 St Andrews Place
Regent's Park
London NW1 4LE
Fax: 020 7487 5218

Index

Page numbers in **bold** refer to tables. Page numbers in *italic* refer to figures.